# CARNIVORE DIET

*A Complete Guide For Carnivores To Lose Weight,Strengthen The Body, Learning The Secret For Best Cooking And The Best Recipes*

By

**ALAN .J. MORRIS**

# TABLE OF CONTENTS

# INTRODUCTION

The globe of food, as well as nutrition, has no absence of charismatic and entertaining characters. At times, I've questioned if this is a relatively new thing born out of the Industrial Transformation's global interruption to food production. At the very least, for the last pair a century, extreme diets combined with severe individualities have usually fit.

Finding a diet plan that benefits you is among one of the most difficult but satisfying difficulties that anybody ever before faces. Whether you're looking to boost your health and wellness, body picture, energy degrees, or relationship with food, there are many different plans to select from. Today, the carnivore diet is acquiring a lot of popularity.

The Carnivore Diet is composed totally of meat and pet products, omitting all other foods.

The diet usually excludes high carbohydrate dairy, so it's a low or absolutely no carbohydrate diet plan. It can be utilized to help reduce weight, reduce inflammation, reverse insulin resistance as well as even more

Fans of the carnivore diet make making a lot of bold wellness asserts regarding this diet. Claims such as boosted skin increased sex drive & muscle mass, far better hormone health and wellness, as well as premium rest top quality.

And also the removal of cravings, autoimmune problems that magically vanish, and a basic consensus that it leaves you looking far better than ever before.

A new diet plan pattern has actually arisen as well as it's obtained the interest of the masses.

The carnivore diet goes completely against the grain of the conventional nutrition guidance we've formerly been educated.

Out of all the fads we have actually been presented to, this diet seems like the most severe one yet.

Yet adhering to a carnivore diet has actually been around for centuries. Our ancestors stuck to a strictly animal-based diet plan, and a few of our longest-living populations grew on carnivore long before "diet plan trends" were ever before introduced.

It's asserted to assist weight-loss, state of mind problems, and also blood sugar regulation, to name a few health concerns. However, the diet plan is exceptionally restrictive and likely unhealthy in the long term. And also, no study backs its purported advantages.

This guide is focused on the human wellness aspects of the diet plan, but it deserves mentioning issues regarding the effects of such a diet plan on the environment. We should focus on human health and wellness. Allowing people to be ill for other pets strikes us as fairly suspicious. That stated we would still like to treat other animals and the atmosphere with as much care as possible. There is no other way for human beings to live without making some impact on their environment. Vegan food derived from mono-crops of soy, wheat, and corn is not sustainable options to meat. They ravage communities and animals residing in them. The good news is, despite popular opinion, livestock production can be compatible with a healthy and balanced world recapturing its atmospheric carbon. Interested visitors must explore alternative management campaigns and also regenerative agriculture for more details. It remains in everybody's best interest to find ways to make the healthiest food in as sustainable a way as feasible. We would certainly constantly advocate for the regard as well as the finest treatment of all living points.

# HISTORY

The diet plan was promoted by Shawn Baker, a former orthopedic specialist based in New Mexico, who published The Carnivore Diet in early 2018. However, in September 2017, his medical permit was revoked by the New Mexico Medical Board, as a result of "failing to report unfavorable action taken by a health care entity as well as inexperience to practice as a licensee."

In recorded history, there are several instances of people from a range of ethnic, cultural and even geographical backgrounds that endured on a meat-centric diet plan as well as remained rather healthy and balanced throughout their lifetime. On the other hand, no civilization has been kept in mind to comply with a simple vegan diet plan with generations. There needs to be a factor behind which lots of people through the ages favored meat as the main component in their diets.

Nowadays, there are many stigmas versus meat. A lot of people appear to be advocating a vegan or vegan and even fruitarian diet plan that is devoid of all meat or animal-sourced food. We are informed that meat is the factor behind artery-blocking, weight gain, high levels of cholesterol, constipation, and so on. Therefore, you must give up meat as well as adhere to a solely plant-based diet plan; however, no human being has individuals who have made it through a healthy diet on a vegan diet from youth till seniority.

If you consider it anthropologically, the real-world examples of different cultures adhering to a specific diet plan are much more legitimate than any kind of clinical research studies that are carried out to recognize something. The truth that people prospered on the carnivore diet via the ages is a much more valid testament that the information collected by clinical research carried out on a couple of people over a few weeks. The former is a much more sensible way of considering the diet plan than the latter, which will certainly involve a team of people consuming more meat than usual for a long time while a study is being performed.

There have been researching studies performed to particularly reveal that a diet plan with fewer animal items is healthier than one with even more of it; however, these research studies have actually mostly failed to show it because a non-vegetarian society is not much less healthy and balanced at all compared to a vegan culture. Animal foods are quite necessary for the health of a human. If you have a look at different groups around the globe and study their history too, you will certainly see that every healthy area makes it through on at least a few animal foods otherwise a whole lot. There is no healthy and balanced group of individuals with full independence from animal-sourced foods.

Like we pointed out prior to 2 particular teams worldwide are used as an archetype of a healthy carnivorous area. The first team is the Eskimos that eat meat and fat virtually exclusively. People who lived in the Arctic areas saw an adjustment in their diet plan just around the latter part of the 1800s when trade routes were being constructed thoroughly. This gave them access to sugar, flour and also other European foods that were then presented into their initial diet; nevertheless, before this adjustment in their diet plan, they were healthier on the diet plan that mostly consisted of animal protein with fat. The second group is the Masai people of Africa who consume really little plant foods and also endure primarily on meat, milk as well as also the blood of animals. The herdsmen from these regions in Africa consumed much more meat when they were age 14-30 considering that these were their warrior years. More meat was considered essential to more powerful bodies and also hence would be valuable for a warrior. It is to be kept in mind though that the old societies that adopted this kind of meat-centric diet did so to adapt to certain extreme ecological elements. A lot of the groups all over the world who adhered to a carnivorous diet stayed in the desert, frozen, or sub-arctic regions. The food is limited in such locations, and also the availability of food is unpredictable as well.

Numerous other neighborhoods survive on a meat-based diet plan also; for instance-- the Inuit of the Canadian Arctic area. Their diet plan is composed mainly of fish, walrus, whale as well as seal meat. In the Russian Arctic, the Chukotka individuals survive on a diet plan of marine animals, caribou meat, and fish. In East Africa, the Samburu, along with the Rendille individuals, have actually endured for several years on a meat and milk diet. In Mongolia, the Steppe nomads generally eat milk items as well as meat daily. In South Dakota, the Sioux are understood to have buffalo meat as the staple in their diet. Beef is almost all of the meals for the Brazilian Gauchos.

As you can see, a meat-eating diet plan has been adhered to throughout the globe for a long time, and these individuals have actually delighted in healthy lives through generations despite the preconception versus meat. The dogma that exists about hydrogenated fat and cholesterol from meat in the American diet plan is completely challenged. The teams of individuals in the Arctic and African people that consume meat loaded diets do not have any taped instances of heart diseases or such disorders in the past, as well as these enhanced only when contemporary foods were presented in their diet plans.

If you take some time to take a look at the diet plan of the ethnic groups that exist in the Arctic region, you will certainly see that they take in hardly any kind of amount of fruit or veggies all year round. Doesn't that make you question how they endure or handle to live healthy lives? You most likely question that they received enough amounts of the important minerals and vitamins in their diet plan after that; nonetheless, they have actually lived such as this for a very long time and prospered on this diet plan as they still do today.

Among the popular researches that sustain the carnivore diet is one performed by a dental expert from Cleveland by the name of Weston A. Rate. He began an examination that he accomplished on the topic for nearly a year. From his occupation, he observed just how the majority of people suffered from oral concerns as well as other metabolic problems. He discovered all the wellness problems and also the facial defects that maintained increasing in the variety of clients he saw. He wondered about the root cause of these problems due to the fact that he thought that God was not the one that would certainly allow this sort of suffering among his people. This curiosity and rate of interest prompted him to investigate the source of all this illness. At that point, 60 years back, there was nobody else that had actually provided this much thought. He was the only one that intended to study various worlds worldwide and also learn the source of the health and wellness problems he discovered in different people. He went from the Swiss area to Africa, Australia and also many more places around the globe. Everything he observed and studied, he wrote in his released publication called "Nourishment as well as Physical Deterioration." This book was quite eye-opening to individuals that review it. Rate's focus got on the food habits of ethnic groups from various parts around the world, which was reasonably unblemished by the contemporary diet. He saw that these people displayed great physical health and wellness and there was hardly any kind of occurrence of the contemporary diseases that are common in the outdoors areas. He was shocked by this and also was curious regarding exactly how they could be in such good health with no help from modern medicine. The essential to all his questions depends on the consuming habits of these separated ethnic groups. His observation was that they all had a diet plan that hardly had any kind of plant fruit and vegetables and was primarily based on animal-sourced products. His study was just another proof of the fact that meat is an extremely healthy component of the human diet plan as well as ought to not be gotten rid of. A meat diet has sufficient quantities of the needed nutrients and minerals that are required for ideal physical wellness.

One more research to be kept in mind is one that was carried out nearly 40 years ago in Point Hope, Alaska. The place is very isolated, as well as this was why they were still on a very meat concentrated diet plan. The research study was published in the year 1972 and also provided different monitorings based on their diet plan and also health and wellness. It stated that the people of Factor Hope were one of the very couples of continuing to the culture that survived on the Eskimo diet plan. Their daily calorie consumption was averaged at 3000 kcal each, and also fifty percent of this was from fat while about 35% was from healthy protein. Only a maximum of 20% of their calories was stemmed from carbohydrates that remained in the kind of pet starch. Their diet plan hardly had any type of grain as well as the only time sucrose was ingested when a little was added to tea or coffee. The research study showed that the locals of Point Hope had virtually 10 times lower occurrence of heart disease compared to the remainder of the general populace in the USA of America. You can see from this that meat does not have a negative effect on your cardiovascular health and wellness, as you are told nowadays. Yet Vilhjalmur Stefansson performed an additional meat-based diet study on the Inuit people in between the years 1906 and 1919. He explained this research in his publication called "The Fat of the Land."

According to this research study, the Inuit eat an entirely meat-based diet plan all the time. Under some rare conditions, they might eat some plant foods like berries, which were protected for eating in the wintertime. If no meat was readily available, they sometimes consumed veggies as a last resource. The anthropologist himself attempted the diet plan for some time however might not stick to it; nonetheless, in his research, he informed of how the Inuit individuals of both genders and all ages were leading healthy thriving lives while enduring on 100% meat. The study additionally said that these individuals were devoid of scurvy and various other meat-related diseases that contemporary civilization fears. They don't also take in any type of salt with their meat yet have no problems associated with salt or electrolyte levels in their body. The research, too, demonstrated just how traditional teams like these thrived on the carnivore diet as well as was in robust health and wellness.

# Carnivore Diet

The carnivore diet plan is likewise called a zero-carb diet plan, carnivorous diet or the all-meat diet plan and has one basic principle; you can only consume meat. Basically, you are meant to consume nearly nothing besides meat for every single solitary dish on a daily basis as long as you are following the diet plan. This diet plan will certainly not determine your portions, calories, food timings or macro percent. You are allowed to consume whenever you are starving and also as much as you require to really feel full. There are certain gray areas that a fan of the diet plan can tailor according to their choice.

As an example, some individuals add components like cream or cheese to their diet while others position a total restriction on consuming anything other than meat. According to the guidelines of the diet plan, you might eat animal-sourced food that consists of meat, eggs or dairy. You can eat as much protein and fat as you should from these foods, yet carbohydrates should be left out from the diet plan.

The carnivore diet is particularly useful due to the carbohydrate-eliminating element. There are specific locations all over the world where people actually survive on no carbs and also instead consume according to the carnivore diet plan. It is not because they are adhering to a fad diet but is a method they have followed for as far back as they can bear in mind. It may sound severe to you when you think of enduring just on meat, fish, and so on with definitely no grains or such carbohydrates. This is primarily since your common diet includes grains as a staple and also you've been informed that they are healthy for your heart. However, the study reveals that the intro of polished carbs is what created a big boost in the rates of diabetes, high blood pressure, tooth cavities, and also atherosclerosis in individuals. This is why a lot of individuals nowadays try removing carbs from their diet plan.

Another major element is that excess carb intake is a significant root cause of weight gain. To be truthful, removing carbs will certainly help some people, while for some, it might not. You can adjust your diet plan as necessary to suit your body's needs. Reducing carbs in your diet plan will certainly aid you in weight-loss and various other health and wellness concerns, yet it is a macro that needs restricting and docsn't constantly require full removal.

Many research studies have been carried out to see the effects of a reduced carbohydrate diet plan on individuals. These reveal that lowering carbs aids to improve mental performance, increase physical endurance, support digestion as well as additionally minimize swelling in the body. A reduced carbohydrate diet plan is also truly great for cardio health and wellness. An additional benefit is that it increases energy while unhealthy food desires are reduced. All these elements together show that the no-carb carnivore diet plan can improve health and also decrease weight also. This diet plan is just among the much more hardcore versions of low-carb or high-fat diet plans like Paleo and Keto diet plans. In this carnivore variation, rather than just reducing carbohydrates, there is total removal of this macro from the diet plan.

The carnivore diet plan has cultural priority as we mentioned earlier. As an example, in Eskimo teams, their diet mainly contained a fish, walrus, or whales as a high-fat pet sourced diet plan. Even in the Masai area of Africa, the diet plan consists majorly of meat with milk. These individuals have actually revealed to have extremely low levels of negative cholesterol and reduced prices of cardiovascular diseases as well.


How to follow the Carnivore Diet

Complying with the diet involves removing all plant foods from your diet plan and solely eating meat, fish, eggs, and also small amounts of low-lactose dairy products.

Foods to consume include beef, hen, pork, lamb, turkey, organ meats, salmon, sardines, white fish, and also percentages of heavy cream and hard cheese. Butter, lard, and bone marrow are additionally enabled.

Supporters of the diet stress eating fatty cuts of meat to reach your everyday power needs.

The Carnivore Diet plan encourages drinking water as well as a bone broth but inhibits drinking tea, coffee, as well as various other beverages made from plants.

It offers no certain guidelines pertaining to calorie consumption, serving dimensions, or how many meals or snacks to eat each day. A lot of proponents of the diet suggest consuming as commonly as you want.

Foods Okay on the Carnivore Diet

Here's what you'll be eating: Red meat (beef, pork, lamb), with an emphasis on fattier cuts of meat to take in enough calories. Other options include:

- Organ meats

- Poultry

- Fish

- Eggs

- Lard

- Bone marrow

- Butter

- Salt and pepper

- Water

- Bone broth

Foods That May Be Okay on the Carnivore Diet

Foods that might be acceptable, as some people interpret the "comes from an animal" part of the carnivore diet, says Schmidt, include:

- Milk

- Yogurt

- Cheese

- Coffee and tea

 These may be plant-based, but some people keep these in the diet.

Foods Not Allowed on the Carnivore Diet

- Vegetables

- Fruit

- Seeds

- Nuts

- Legumes

- Bread

- Pasta

- Grains

# 30-Days Carnivore Diet Meal Plan (Menus, Recipes & Shopping Lists)

OK, so you're still with us, as well as you've made a note of your goals and also establish a timeline to get going.

Currently, it's time to assist you out and also intend your meat intake for each day of the week. I'll provide out an everyday dish plan based upon breakfast lunch as well as dinner, along with the quantities you'll need.

This is based on a typical height as well as a size person, yet if you have extreme weight-loss or muscle gain goals, then you will require to readjust these.

Also, if you discover you're still hungry after consuming these sections, then boost the quantities gradually.


Shopping list for the week:

- Bacon: 12 ounces

- 100% pork sausages: 13 ounces

- Pork chops: 12 ounces

- Pork belly: 10 ounces

- Lamb Chops: 24 ounces

- Chicken breasts

- Ground beef: 18 ounces

- Porterhouse steak: 24 ounce

- Ribeye steak: 24 ounce

- Topside of beef 24 ounces

- Salmon cutlets: 30 ounces

- Trout: 26 ounces

- Butter: 1lbs

- Cheese: 1/2 lbs

Week 2 Diet Plan and Shopping List

This week, we're mosting likely to be getting rid of a lot of the dairy products. We'll still enable some butter to be used in cooking, but the celebrity is gone now.

I would also suggest that you begin trying out a little with the way you prepare your meats. For the beef, try and transfer to the uncommon side of cooking as this will maintain a great deal of the nutritional values.

The more you cook something, the more of the protein, minerals, and vitamins break down. We'll still be maintaining a mix of seafood, poultry, pork, lamb, as well as beef, yet we'll additionally add in somebody organ meat also.

Some people are a bit squeamish about this, yet if you search for the nutrients they include, you might change your mind.

You can additionally ask your butcher to reduce them into slices.

Shopping list for the week:

- Chicken breasts: 32 ounces

- Topside of beef: 44 ounces

- Lamb chops: 12 ounces

- Salmon cutlets: 30 ounces

- Ribeye steak: 28 ounces

- Ribeye steak: 24 ounce

- 100% pork sausages: 3 ounces

- Porterhouse steak: 12 ounces

- Pork chops: 12 ounces

- Beef liver: 12 ounces

Week 3 Diet Plan and Shopping List

OK, this week, we're getting rid of all the milk items left as well as we'll somewhat boost the change towards beef.

You'll see that there are less dishes covered by fish and also poultry and we'll also add in a beef-only day to prepare for next week.

At this phase, you need to additionally be consuming your beef at least tool to get most of the micronutrient benefits. You will have prepared a great deal of beef and also must be obtaining used to judging it much bettcr.

What you can additionally do is cut your steaks in half and then cook one part medium-rare and also the various other medium-well. One thing you should discover is that there is a whole lot even more flavor to the medium-rare part.

I'm also introducing a little bit of extra organ meat into the mix. These are very beneficial to stabilize your efforts, although they are lower in fats.

From one serving of liver or kidney, you can obtain more than your everyday demand of Vitamin B, consisting of B12.

Shopping list for the week:

- Chicken breasts: 12 ounces

- Topside of beef: 36 ounces

- Lamb chops: 8 ounces

- Salmon cutlets: 15 ounces

- Ribeye steak: 24 ounces

- Bacon: 4 ounces

- 100% pork sausages: 3 ounces

- Porterhouse steak: 32 ounces

- Beef liver: 8 ounces

- Beef Kidney: 8 ounces

Week 4 Diet Plan and Shopping List

If you have actually made it this far, then you can start anticipating truly discovering some benefits.

You should be really feeling a whole lot extra physical and also mental power as a result of your metabolism, having actually fully changed to ketosis.

You ought to also find those carb yearnings will have lowered because you're currently a lot better equipped to obtain all the energy you need from fat.

Today, we'll be getting rid of all meat that does not come from cows. You'll also observe that we include body organ meat on a much more normal basis. As well as there is another point that you need to attempt and factor in for this week.

All the meat you acquire ought to come from grass-fed only cows. It does not have to be natural. However, that is an alternative if you can manage it. If your budget does not extend to this, then try as well as add in as much grass-fed as feasible.

Also, due to the fact that there really aren't any kind of dishes to comply with on a meat-only diet plan, you must try and vary your cooking strategies. I find barbecuing your meat is a wonderful way to get some of the charred tastes.

Shopping list for the week:

- Topside of beef: 36 ounces

- Ground beef: 56 ounces

- Ribeye steak: 28 ounces

- Porterhouse steak: 32 ounces

- Beef liver: 8 ounces

Monday

- Breakfast: eggs, bacon, sardines

- Lunch: turkey burger patty, salmon jerky, beef tips

- Dinner: filet mignon, crab, chicken liver

- Snacks: a small amount of Parmesan cheese, jerky

Tuesday

- Breakfast: shrimp, eggs, a small glass of heavy cream

- Lunch: strip steak, tuna fish, beef jerky

- Dinner: Lamb chops, scallops, beef liver

- Snacks: a small amount of hard Cheddar cheese, bone broth

Wednesday

- Breakfast: eggs, salmon, turkey sausage

- Lunch: beef tips, pork chops, mackerel

- Dinner: turkey burger patty, a small amount of Parmesan cheese, bone marrow

- Snacks: hard-boiled eggs, shrimp

Thursday

- Breakfast: trout, shredded chicken, bacon

- Lunch: beef meatballs, small amount Cheddar cheese, salmon jerky

- Dinner: crab cooked in lard, filet mignon

- Snacks: sardines, beef jerky

Friday

- Breakfast: eggs, chicken and turkey sausage links

- Lunch: lamb roast, chicken liver, pork chop

- Dinner: flank steak, scallops cooked in butter, a small glass of heavy cream

- Snacks: bone broth, turkey jerky

Meals and snacks on the Carnivore Diet consist entirely of animal products and offer little variety.

23

A carnivorous diet plan is not simply tough because of the conversations with vegans that always appear to wind up with you being compared to a mass murderer.

Yet, when you make a radical change in what you consume, then tiny mistakes can end up minimizing your success price. Below are a couple of a lot more pointers to help set you up for the most effective outcomes.

1. Check Out The Fatty Cuts

Discover The Fatty Cuts

When I first began, I believed I was doing myself support by only getting lean cuts of meat.

Nevertheless, once your body switches over to ketosis, you will certainly need a lot of fat in your diet plan as a resource of energy.

Just how much will certainly very much depend on your day-to-day activity.

If you have a physical job and head to the gym consistently, after that, you'll require a whole lot more than if your day focuses on bed, auto, lift, desk, lift, cars and truck, sofa, and also back to bed.

## 2. Come to be More Energetic

Come to be a lot more energetic

Occupying running or swimming or going to the health club more than once a week is vital to your overall health and wellness.

And also, if you have specific fat burning objectives, after that, you have to place your muscular tissues and metabolic rate under some pressure.

In the first couple of days as well as weeks, this will likewise aid in removing any excess glucose as well as glycogen, which will reduce the amount of keto-flu symptoms.

## 3. Do not Be Too Concerned About Calories

Don't Be As Well Worried Regarding Calories

Yes, I did claim that yet if you integrate a really active life with an all-meat diet plan, after that, it's instead not likely that you'll remain in a considerable state of calorie overdose.

As well as that, due to the fact that the calories are not coming from carbohydrates, you won't be keeping them as fat.

What will actually take place is that if you consume a lot more fat than your body needs, it will go through undigested.

Not to appear as well revolting, but keep an eye out for indicators of looseness of the bowels to aid you to tweak your meals.

4. Keep A Food Journal

Maintain a food journal

Nutritional macros like protein will be available in abundance, as well as undoubtedly, and carbs are a no-go nutrient.

However, one of the most significant troubles you can experience is generally down to the micro-nutrients you require.

Finding the correct amounts of vitamins, minerals, as well as electrolytes, is exceptionally essential.

That's why you require to revolve in between various cuts of meat as well as include organ meat also.

You can take some supplements on the carnivore diet, including mineral and vitamin tablets, and also do not hesitate to include some salt to your food. It will be crucial to maintaining your moistened.

# Getting Through The First Month Of An All-Meat Diet

Before you dive right into the carnivore diet plan, it is very important to know that the very first month and particularly the very first week will be the hardest.

Below are a few things you should recognize and also incorporate to make the change easier:

•        Obtain your blood examined. Get your blood work done prior to you start the carnivore diet plan and also again after around 2 months in. Everyone has various metabolic requirements, so it's important to understand whether the diet plan is functioning well with your body.

•        Don't stop when you do not really feel good. You'll greater than most likely experience tiredness, headaches, and other flu-like signs during the very first week of the diet plan. This is a typical part of the process as your body is getting made use to using fats for power rather than carbohydrates.

•        Your cravings will rise and fall. You'll have some days where you want to consume non-stop and various other days where you won't also consider food. Your hunger will certainly change as soon as your body gets utilized in this way of consuming.

Does Carnivore Cause Vitamin C Deficiencies (Scurvy)?

You might have heard that carnivore can trigger scurvy-- a condition that causes a variety of symptoms from completely dry skin as well as hair to shed teeth.

Scurvy was common with pirates and also seafarers before the 18th century. They would go out to sea with just jerky to eat, as well as the lack of fresh vegetables and fruits would diminish their vitamin C stores, eventually causing their teeth, skin, and nails to develop sores.

Vitamin C is water-soluble, and dehydrating meat removes vitamin C web content. Nevertheless, fresh meat does include a percentage of vitamin C, specifically, if the meat is grass-fed [*]

On top of that, individuals on a low-carb diet really have higher vitamin C degrees (and also other antioxidant degrees) than individuals on a higher-carb diet do, recommending that you either ended up being more reliable at using vitamin C or you call for much less of it when you aren't eating carbs [*]

If you're still worried, you can constantly take a vitamin C supplement. Regarding 1000 mg of vitamin C a day is ample to keep scurvy at bay.

Does Carnivore Work for Athletes?

There's no research study on carnivore for professional athletes, yet a lot of individuals report succeeding in the health club when they're on a carnivore.

That said, if you locate you're shedding endurance in the gym after the first few weeks of a carnivore, you may wish to add in some carbohydrates, or try a basic keto diet.

If that still does not seem like enough, you can try a targeted ketogenic diet plan or cyclical ketogenic diet plan.

Does Carnivore Cause Nutrient Deficiencies

There's not much great research on whether or not an all-meat diet plan will certainly trigger nutrient deficiencies.

You will not fulfill all your suggested everyday consumption (RDIs) of nutrients on an all-meat diet. Nonetheless, your nutrient needs might also alter when you stop refining carbs [*]

A growing variety of people report no nutrient deficiencies in their blood work, even after months to years of eating just meat. Red meat consists of lots of (however not all) vitamins, minerals, as well as various other trace elements, especially if the meat is from a grass-fed animal.


Carnivore diet vs. Low Carb and Keto

The carnivore diet plan does overlap-- yet very little-- with a ketogenic, paleo or low carb diets.

Indeed, a carnivore diet plan makes the carbohydrate restrictions of also the keto diet plan look rather mild!

While keto and also similar diets are high protein and fat with some carbs, the carnivore diet plan consists virtually solely of healthy protein as well as fat.

Keto now has a reasonable and expanding body of research study behind it. On the other hand, the carnivore diet, save the earlier work entailing Steffenson, hasn't been researched a lot. Therefore, not much research study feeds on how to establish proportions of fat to protein, and so on to offer you advice.

The only exception to the carbohydrate intake is if you consume fresh dairy. Fresh and also some fermented milk products can include a reasonable amount of carbs (unless the whey is removed a la Greek yogurt). Some carnivores welcome them while others do not.

For those on this diet plan, it is essential to embrace a nose to tail strategy to eating, balancing muscular tissue meat with the remainder of the pet and the pet's products-- consisting of eggs and also milk. If this is not done, the carnivore diet plan will certainly be harmful as opposed to the healing experience.

What are the downsides to going on the Carnivore Diet

Well, it can not be all good ...

While it holds true that the Carnivore Diet plan is showing unbelievably prominent today, there are constantly posting likely to be disadvantages to a nutritional program that radically transforms your diet, which is going to hold true unless your basic everyday wish list currently looks like a carnivore Diet plan food list.

Before saying anything else, allow's address the massive, roaring, the elephant in the room...

Restrictive diet plans are extremely challenging to stick to in the long-term!

Yes, there will be success stories and also star recommendations. Yes, there are undeniable benefits to inspire you to stay with the diet.

Yet remember, a star or elite degree-professional athlete has the time to dedicate themselves to sticking to this diet plan. You on the other hand, being as you are a plain mortal like the rest of us, will certainly have to balance consuming a restrictive diet plan with tasks, family members dedications, and also life.

Instantly, steak for breakfast every morning may not seem so attractive when you've slept in, and also, you're late for work ...

Perhaps unsurprisingly, like all trending diets, the Carnivore Diet plan has additionally been met with strong opposition, in addition to passionate assistance.

Wealth in meat = deficiencies in other places

Several critics of the diet plan say that consuming simply meat will certainly cause deficiencies in particular areas of your diet plan. Nonetheless, of the existing research study relating to meat consumption, the number of researches associating with physically active individuals is infrequent.

Be tired with your option of meat (within your budget plan).

Some red meat has actually been discovered to have actually added hormonal agents, which have been connected to breast cancer cells, so stick to natural where possible.

This will, naturally, be identified by accessibility, in addition to your budget plan. Nonetheless, when in doubt, additionally try and also guide away from mass-produced meat and also circumstances where you can't recognize the origin of the meat.


Social Disadvantages

There are possible social disadvantages to the Carnivore Diet plan, also.

When heading out to consume with your good friends, it may be a problem when it concerns the food selection, especially if the location you have actually selected is very carb-heavy, or lacking in fresh cuts of meat. Nevertheless, it is additionally reasonable to point out that the majority of restaurants will possibly be able to aid you out with the matter, as well as will certainly be able to accommodate your needs.

If you are most likely to handle the Carnivore Diet over time, you need to additionally think of whether it'll damage your wallet or handbag. Nevertheless, as the fitness supplement sector is expanding, there are places where you can obtain cheaper organic/ clean meat.

## BENEFITS

While the concept of eating as much meat as you like absolutely interest the palate. However, as holds true with any type of recommended diet plan, it is very important to understand as well as value the effects it will carry your health. Nevertheless, there is a reason why your present nourishment plan isn't working, as well as knowing whether the brand-new one will combat those issues is essential.

Below are the crucial health advantages that can be given by buying the carnivore diet.

## WEIGHT LOSS

Losing weight is the most typical resource of motivation for beginning any kind of diet, and decreasing your carb consumption is just one of the quickest routes to success. We've all heard the "no carbohydrates before carbs" concept and also, while

41

it's not straight connected to the carnivore diet plan, its beliefs prove out.

Reduced carbohydrate diets such as the carnivore diet motivate quick weight-loss. There are a number of factors for this, consisting of but not limited to:

•        Protein as well as fat leaves you are feeling fuller for longer (contrasted to carbs), implying you are much less likely to eat way too much and eat extreme calories-- consisting of snacks in between meals.

•        Feeling satiated lowers circumstances of snacking because of monotony or tension.

•        The carnivore diet motivates paying attention to the body's natural cravings indications, which makes dieting a whole lot much easier from a motivational degree due to the lack of cravings or shame from calorie counting.

Numerous researches have revealed a correlation between high-protein, low-carb diets, and considerable weight loss that can be maintained.


The human body flourishes on healthy proteins and fats, which can likewise offer boosted power levels for physical activities.

To recognize just how the carnivore diet plan works for fat burning, we need to take a birds-eye view of just how weight loss functions as well as what components comprise an efficient weight management plan.

At its core, excess energy is saved as body fat as well as excessive body-fat is normally the outcome of a long term calorie excess - which implies spending a large amount of time-consuming extra food than your body usually melts in a day.

According to a scientist named Max Wishnofsky, we can presume that:

- One extra pound equals 454 grams.

- Pure fat has 8.7-- 9.5 calories per gram.

- Body fat cells are 87% fat.

Using those worths, we can wrap up that a pound of body fat actually includes anywhere from 3,436 to 3,752 calories.

HOW IT WORKS

Prepared for some scientific research? To recognize how weight management works, as well as what elements comprise weight-loss, we need to check out overall day-to-day energy expenses (TDEE). Your

TDEE is the number of calories your body expends or utilizes each day. To understand exactly how this works much better, let's damage the 4 aspects of what TDEE is comprised of:


Total Daily Energy Expenditure


Each of the components is composed of a different percent of TDEE, which is shown in the diagram above. Allow's damage these parts down:

Rested Power Expenditure (REE).

•        Basal metabolic price (BMR) - BMR is the number of calories your body burns each day whilst relaxing. If you were to depend on a bed as well as do no task all day, this is the number of calories your body burns. This is a type of REE or relaxed power expenditure.

Non-Rested Power Expense (NREE).

•        Non-Exercise Task Thermogenesis (NEAT) - NEAT is how many calories your body burns daily whilst doing general activities. This might entail points like walking, cleaning, and carrying shopping bags residence from a grocery store.

•	Exercise Task Thermogenesis (EAT) - This is the number of calories you expend through planned exercise, like weight training, running, dancing, and so forth.

•	Thermic Impact of Food (TEF) - This is how many calories your body uses up through absorbing foods.

For fat loss, the most important thing is to achieve a calorie deficiency.

This can be achieved in two methods:

•	Increasing EAT as well as NEAT by moving more each day.

•	A calorie deficit is via a nutrition protocol.

Creating a dietary calorie shortage ought to be the foundation of all fat loss diet plans no matter whether you choose carnivore, periodic fasting, or any other preferred nutrition method.

## BENEFITS OF THE CARNIVORE DIET FOR WEIGHT LOSS

Eating a carnivore diet plan will create you to lose fat, yet only if you can achieve a calorie shortage. Nonetheless, any kind of diet plan where a calorie shortage is produced will create you to lose fat. So what makes the carnivore diet plan various? And also, why would certainly you pick to go carnivore instead of going with various other preferred nutrition procedures?

Because like our ancestors, you are only eating animal products as well as not consuming carbs. This triggers your body to enter into "ketosis." Ketosis is a state in which your body breaks down fat cells as well as creates molecules called ketones. Rather than running on carbohydrates, your body utilizes ketones for gas.

We have broken down all the health and wellness advantages of the carnivore diet plan formerly, yet exactly how specifically can the carnivore diet plan advantage those intended to shed fat?


Increased Energy

Whilst it may take numerous months to become adjusted to a reduced carb, high-fat diet plan (LCHF), a research study was conducted to figure out whether marathon runners had the ability to adjust to it without an impediment to efficiency. According to Chang, Borer and also Lin, it might in fact improve efficiency. High carbohydrate foods launch cost-free tryptophan, which creates fatigue and tiredness. Carnivore has zero carbohydrates - so integrated with your body being in ketosis, and we can see why so many individuals that comply with the carnivore dit report a rise in energy.

Less Hunger

According to Gibson et alia, who carried out an organized evaluation and meta-analysis of ketogenic diets on hunger levels, people who adhere to a ketogenic diet plan were much less hungry as well as had much less wish to consume. It deserves stating that the studies evaluated were in the context of energy limitation, or a calorie deficit, so it is very pertinent to fat burning. As carnivore places you right into ketosis, it needs to make cravings a lot more manageable.

Mental Clarity

Whilst numerous diets can leave you really feeling low power as well as weary, there are numerous accounts in on the internet carnivore neighborhoods of individuals having more psychological clarity. This is most likcly to be triggered by a boost in healthy protein. A study conducted by Jakobsen et alia, showed a high healthy protein diet plan enhanced response time as well as cognitive function, contrasted to a modest healthy protein team.

Thermic Effect of Food

Out of all the macronutrients (fats, carbohydrates as well as healthy protein), the one that takes one of the most energy to absorb is protein. Getting on carnivore means you'll be melting even more calories without doing anything. Why does this issue? Because of the parts of energy expense is TEF or the thermic effect of food. It may only account for a small number of additional calories shed each day, but in time this builds up, assisting add to weight-loss.

# HOW TO WORK OUT YOUR CALORIES FOR WEIGHT LOSS ON CARNIVORE

A lot of individuals begin complying with the carnivore diet plan for fat loss and do not track calories - and also, they still lose body-fat. That being stated, we advise having an understanding of how to calculate your calorie demands so you don't over-consume by chance.

The math is a bit complicated, so we've additionally consisted of a calculator listed below. We utilize the Modified Harris-Benedict Equation:

- Men BMR = 88.362 + (13.397 x weight in kg) + (4.799 x elevation in centimeters) - (5.677 x age in years).

- Ladies BMR = 447.593 + (9.247 x weight in kg) + (3.098 x height in cm) - (4.330 x age in years).


## HOW TO MEASURE PROGRESS

Measuring progression is extremely crucial in a fat loss diet plan. Among the main reasons tracking progress is so vital, is due to the fact that if weight management stalls, you can deal with the factor early on as well as make changes to your calorie intake. Tracking development typically revolves around 3 points - dimensions, body weight, and progression pictures.

This can be done regular or regular monthly as well as right here's exactly how to do it:

•       Chest: Place one end of the tape measure at the max part of your bust, wrap it around (under your underarms, around your shoulder blades, and back to the front).

•       Arm: Cover the measuring tape around the widest part of your arm from front to back as well as around to the start point.

•       Waistline: Use the tape to circle your midsection over your stubborn belly switch and below your chest without sucking in your belly.

•       Hips: Make sure the tape mores than the biggest part of your buttocks.

•       Upper leg: Wrap the measuring tape around the maximum location of your thigh from front to back. You may be attracted to rip off by reducing the tape measure a couple of inches, but then you won't obtain an exact measurement.

In addition to this, taking a weekly or daily dimension of your body weight is also a great suggestion. The best time to gauge your body weight is the first point in the morning after using the washroom and also before eating food or water to make sure uniformity.

Ultimately, dimensions are excellent due to the fact that sometimes, your body weight can remain the same for an extended period of time. That may mean you're developing muscle whilst shedding body fat, so seeing your waist go down but bodyweight remains the same ways you get on the appropriate track. Using a tape measure, take measurements of your shoulders, waist, hips, arms as well as quads.

INCLUDE EXERCISE

Keep in mind the elements that makeup energy expenses? EAT as well as NEAT, do compose a percentage of the amount of calories your body burns. If you consider the portions, NEAT really composes a much larger percentage of calories shed compared to CONSUME.

That suggests that merely by being much more energetic every day, you in fact end up shedding more calories than going to the gym every day. Doing points like routine vigorous walking, yoga as well as even cycling to function will certainly help you accomplish greater degrees of NEAT. Some individuals are doing the carnivore diet for weight loss select to do some weight training to assist build and/or keep muscle mass. This is really helpful for weight-loss, yet it is not extremely important to your success.

# DIABETES CONTROL

While (as already mentioned), any person taking medication for diabetic issues should stay clear of the diet plan or at the very least get in touch with a doctor, the carnivore diet plan can proactively support the battle against both Type 1 as well as Type 2 diabetes mellitus. It is shown to assist the management of Kind 1 while it can possibly turn around Type 2 entirely.

The carnivore diet plan's absence of carbohydrates, as well as fine-tuned sugars, helps support blood glucose levels. Blood sugar level degrees will not endure the big spikes that consuming cookies, bread, pasta, and other high-carb foods generate, ultimately resulting in a far smaller (or potentially no) reliance on insulin and also other monitoring techniques.

In addition to combating existing signs of Type 1 and Kind 2 diabetes, the application of a carnivore diet plan can help stop the very early threats becoming diabetic issues whether a preventative tool or a management one, the prospective to combat diabetes is a major favorable.

# IRRITABLE BOWEL SYNDROME (IBS)

Irritable Digestive tract Syndrome, otherwise understood merely as IBS, can take numerous forms. The signs and symptoms include discomfort as well as pain in the gut typically qualified by gas, bloating, diarrhea, and aches. IBS can additionally prompt acid indigestion, reflux, and also a range of various other problems relating to the digestion system. Changing to the carnivore diet plan can help in reducing or remove the signs and symptoms.

This is because of most of IBS symptoms surface area (or at the minimum become substantially more noticeable) due to planting food usage. Grains, legumes, and other ingredients that the body doesn't absorb are usually the perpetrators. The carnivore diet plan stays clear of those potentially damaging foods, suggesting it can be the ideal diet plan for dealing with IBS.

The carnivore diet does not actively get rid of the tummy or gastrointestinal system's sensitivity to gluten as well as other substances. Nevertheless, the truth that you will not be exposed to the troublesome materials makes it seem like a remedy.

## EPILEPSY MANAGEMENT

Low-carb diet plans have been made use of to combat epilepsy for nearly a century, as well as the intro of a carnivore diet plan can bring those advantages also. Initially utilized to treat children, low and no-carb diet plans are now recognized as an appropriate administration procedure for grown-up sufferers also.

It is shown that carnivore diet plans can reduce the frequency of seizures, which can allow patients to enjoy the rewards of needing fewer medicines and drugs in their fight to handle the problem. Provided the many adverse effects credited to epilepsy monitoring drugs, such as personality changes as well as reduced concentration levels, this is considered a really favorable end result.

Some followers of the carnivore diet plan have actually even reported to damage cost-free entirely from the reliance or usage of epilepsy drugs. Nonetheless, also those that still require them often discover that the regularities are considerably reduced.


## POLY-CYSTIC OVARY SYNDROME (PCOS)

PCOS, which represents Poly-cystic ovary syndrome, is a problem that impacts over 1 in 10 females. It can cause menstrual issues, a range of physical pains, acne, excessive weight, and also make a woman infertile. It is connected to insulin resistance and Kind 2 diabetes mellitus, which is just one of the reasons why the carnivore diet plan can be associated with efficient monitoring.

Also, the weight-loss qualities of the carnivore diet plan can sustain customers in the fight versus PCOS. The included advantages of leveled hormonal agents, blood glucose levels, and lowered insulin needs can all feed right into the suggestion of combatting PCOS. Several research studies have highlighted a link between low-carb as well as no-carb diets with turning around PCOS, making it possible for individuals to lead a less disrupted way of livings and also even fall pregnant.

# STRENGTHEN THE BODY

The carnivore diet plan is an excellent suggestion for bodybuilders due to the fact that it gives huge volumes of protein, vitamins, and minerals.

At the same time, it tons you up with lots of energy to power through your training.

If you take a gradual approach to switch your diet plan away from plants as well as towards only meat, then you need to notice a matching shift in how much more physical power and also endurance you have available.

Currently, this is a lifestyle choice that will raise a few brows, yet when you can demonstrate results via raised muscular tissue mass and also strength, you'll quickly place the movie critics in their location.

Assuming you have actually provided your body the needed time to adapt to the Carnivore Diet plan and also get to a homeostatic collection factor.

Currently, you certainly will need to have some really intense exercises and toughness training program in place, yet if you're really looking to bulk up, after that, you have to pay a lot of attention to what and also just how much you eat.

Let's go through how to build muscle on the carnivore diet.

Work Out Your Calorie Needs

When you intend a diet to get mass muscle weight, all of it boils down to calories. The typical healthy and balanced grownup will certainly require about 2,000 calories a day, yet during a bulking stage, that will certainly require to enhance dramatically.

You should never depend on your cravings, as you'll need to eat greater than you require to sustain muscle growth.

Expert professional athletes who invest 4 or even more hours working out will certainly commonly take in 2 or more times the day-to-day average.

Vary The Meats You Consume

There is no person finest meat for bodybuilding, however, one point to avoid is the really lean cuts that have little to no fat. On the meat-only diet plan, you will require all the power from fat to sustain your toughness training.

When it pertains to finding out what to consume for muscular tissue gain, I typically aim for great deals of beef and also chicken as it gives a great mix of fat and healthy protein. Throw in some fish for some additional trace elements, and also, you'll have all feasible health facets covered.

Time Your Meals Precisely

A weight lifting diet to get muscle mass isn't nearly what you eat, but when you eat your food too. As meat, as well as fat, take longer to digest than carbohydrates, you have to plan the meals a little bit extra.

This is not as important for cardio training, however when you're heading to the fitness center to raise heavyweights, then purpose to eat around 60 to 90 minutes before.

Take Regular Off Cycles

The very best recommendations I got when I started was that a carnivore diet plan for constructing muscle mass is not something you ought to do lasting. I usually go for 6 to 10-week cycles, as well as the time these with the major bulking workouts.

You'll still be able to get the majority of your amino acids and also power from the food you consume during off-cycles, yet you'll also have some even more flexibility when it concerns carbs as well as supplements like whey as well as creatine.

Supplements Should You Take

However, there have actually been researches that revealed the specific contrary to be the situation. Now, if you do end up constipated, after that, you can definitely check out some fiber supplements, whether it's carnivore diet plan weight reduction or bulking that you're going for.

Simply keep one point in mind. Your gastrointestinal system is incredibly efficient at breaking down and soaking up meat, along with all the fat, amino acids, vitamins, and minerals.

This means really little waste is left, and what some people wrap up as being irregularity, can typically be simply much less waste to poop out.

One more type of supplement you most likely have actually taken previously is post-exercise drinks to assist with muscle healing. I still take these myself. However, you have to beware of the active ingredients to ensure they aren't loaded with carbohydrates.

# NUTRITIONAL BENEFITS

Meat obtains quite lousy press coverage in general, whether it's for obvious wellness or ecological reasons. You can certainly make great debates on the honest side of things, yet when done right, consuming meat can provide substantial wellness benefits.

In this section, I want to concentrate a lot more on the dietary values of fat, carbohydrates, as well as healthy protein, so that you can attempt and also intend your food intake a bit much better to take full advantage of calories as well as macros.

Here is what percent of weight makes up fat and protein.

Beef

- Fat: In between 20% and also 30% for the majority of hamburger and ribeye cuts

- Protein: Between 30% and 40% for ribeye and also round steak

The outright top suggestion for bodybuilders is beef, as it loads a lot of calories and an outstanding mix between fat and healthy protein. It's quite very easy to switch over in between various cuts throughout the day to either obtain more fat or a lot more protein.

Additionally, because you can prepare it even more to the rare end of the range, you'll protect a great deal more of the amino acids without breaking them down with sustained high warm. That's one of the most substantial advantages over all other types detailed here.

Pork

Fat: 10% to 15% depending on the preparation approach

Healthy protein: Concerning 25% for the average pork chop

Pork has a respectable percent of healthy protein. However, you have to account for a few of that healthy protein degenerating throughout the food preparation procedure. On the fat side of points, you can get a tasty pork stubborn belly cut, yet again, a great deal of the fat will certainly melt as well as melt away throughout the preparation.

Lamb

- Fat: 15% for the ordinary lamb chop

- Healthy protein: Between 30% and 40% usually

Lamb is fairly high in protein, and because you can slow down prepare it at low warmth, and also offer it even more to the unusual end of the range, you will not lose too much of the nutritional worth. Fat is additionally reasonably high, but this does rely on the cut you choose.

The large disadvantage of lamb is the cost. Compared to beef, you will certainly be paying a premium, as well as taking into consideration the quantity, and you'll require to eat, this can add up quickly.

Chicken

- Fat: Reduced 3% for poultry breast and also concerning 10% for thighs

- Protein: Between 25% and 30%, varying between breast and thighs

A hen is a large favorite among all sorts of professional athletes since it's stuffed filled with protein. And the kind of healthy protein is very easily absorbed. However, on the fat side of points, it's very reduced, and also the food preparation process will remove a lot of it.

Fish & Fish and shellfish

- Fat: Generally below 5% fat

- Healthy protein: Usually, just above 20%.

The factor for adding fish as well as fish and shellfish to your diet is to get all the health advantages of the Omega Fatty Acids in addition to numerous nutrients.

It's not the most loading if you need to consume huge quantities of different foods, but adding some to your dish plan on a regular basis is still a great concept.

It's clear that muscle-building needs a great deal of healthy protein that you would normally get from meat, eggs, and specific types of beans. But you can achieve so much extra in much less time, by changing totally to meat.

## COMMON MISTAKES ON THE CARNIVORE DIET

- Consuming too little food (this causes undesirable too much weight management or other symptoms).

- Not drinking enough water (drink to please thirst and prevent dehydration).

- Not adding salt to food (you can experience the same keto flu signs and symptoms on this diet plan too).

- Consuming a moderate all-meat diet plan with added fruits, vegetables & other kinds of carbohydrates.

- Preventing fatty meats (don't fear the cholesterol is good for you).

What to Stay clear of on the Carnivore Diet plan.

At first, we wish to keep the diet plan as easy as possible so you can reach a great baseline.

Prevent the following:

- Anything that's not meat or salt.

- Vegetable oils.

- Initially, don't eat poultry. The fat, as well as nutrient profile, is inferior to the other options above.

- Veggies.

- Sauces.

- Carbohydrates.

- Supplements.

- Refined meats: They contain way too many ingredients Keep an eye out for nitrates and also nitrites and also prevent them.

- No delicious dark chocolate initially. Sorry.

- Bitching as well as groaning.

Wait, vegetables? Yes, you check out that right. Veggies are packed with endogenous chemicals that can irritate you. Unpleasant compounds like oxalates, which can trigger kidney stones. Goitrogens which damage your thyroid. As well as lectins that ruin your digestive tract.

The goal is to eliminate as long as possible, then do a controlled test by including back later to see if you can tolerate it.

# HOW TO COOK YOUR MEAT

Cooking? That's for modernized losers?

Yes, some people do eat raw. Yet that's not what I advise.

There are numerous alternatives for how to prepare your meat — Cook to your very own preference.

However, you ought to make sure not to overcook your food. Treat your steak with love as well as treatment. You want your steak to remain juicy when it's completed.

If you overcook your food, you can decrease the nutrient content. The adhering to nutrients are often reduced throughout cooking:

- Water-soluble vitamins: Vitamin C as well as the B vitamins

- Fat-soluble vitamins: Vitamins A, D, E, and also K.

- Minerals: Largely potassium, magnesium, salt and also calcium

# Carnivore Diet Food List

If you have actually reached the stage of dedicating to the carnivore diet, then creating a food list of meat-based products is essential.

We know that starting a brand-new diet is discouraging, let alone substantially changing exactly how you approach food. Our Carnivore Diet Food List is consequently created to be dealt with as a wish list: what you require to begin on the Carnivore Diet immediately!

Compared to other consuming patterns and fad diets, the carnivore diet food selection is pretty straight-forward. Meat, fish, chicken, eggs, and also specific milk products are enabled, and most various other foods should be gotten rid of.

- Meat: beef, pork, lamb, veal, bison, offal

- Fish and shellfish: salmon, tuna, mackerel, anchovies, codfish

- Poultry: hen, turkey, goose, duck

- Eggs and also egg whites

- Milk Products: low-lactose foods like hard cheeses and also butter

- Beverages: water, bone brew

Below are several of the ingredients that ought to stay clear of as part of the diet plan:

- Fruits: apples, bananas, oranges, berries, pears, peaches, plums

- Veggies: broccoli, cauliflower, spinach, kale, zucchini, tomatoes, bell peppers

- Legumes: chickpeas, kidney beans, black beans, lentils, pinto beans

- Nuts: almonds, walnuts, macadamia nuts, pecans, cashews, pistachios

- Seeds: chia seeds, flax seeds, pumpkin seeds, hemp seeds, sunflower seeds

- Grains: amaranth, quinoa, wheat, buckwheat, rice, oats, barley, pasta

- Dairy products Products: high-lactose foods like milk, yogurt, and soft cheeses

- Refined foods: chips, biscuits, cookies, candy, ease meals, convenience food

- Beverages: tea, coffee, sports beverages, soft drinks, energy drinks

- Sugars: table sugar, brownish sugar, honey, maple syrup

## SHOPPING LIST

Meat, cheese, eggs, and full-fat milk/heavy lotion.

However, there are some things which you could not at first think about putting onto your grocery store list that is actually pretty good to have. Whilst these could sound a little unattractive, the health advantages are unsurpassed.

Organ meats include points such as liver, heart, as well as kidneys. They contain wonderful nutrients, such as folate, iron, zinc, and also selenium.

Bone marrow the within bones, in charge of creating blood, teems with an omega-3 fatty acid, jelly, and also collagen, which are wonderful for you. Whilst you can roast and also divided open a bone to get at the spongy goodness within, you can also obtain benefits of consuming bone marrow by consuming bone broth.

Many also fail to remember that oily fish are likewise excellent carnivore diet plan food. It s not all steak and ribs, you recognize. Again, these are a great source of omega-3 fatty acid, minerals, and also vitamins that will certainly maintain you healthy whilst on the diet plan. So, don t forget to add those to your checklist, also.

Meat

Beef.

- Bone Marrow.

- Chicken.

- Body organ meat.

- Mind.

- Heart.

- Kidneys.

- Liver.

- Lungs.

- Tongue.

- Pork.

- Turkey.


- Milk & Eggs.

- Butter.

- Cheese.

- Eggs.

- Heavy cream/full-fat milk.

- Flavoring.

- Salt.

- Drinks.

- Bone brew.

Water.


Fish & Shellfish.

- Cod.

- Herring.

- Haddock.

- Mackerel.

- Oysters.

- Salmon.

- Shrimp.

- Whitebait.

If your taste is salivating, and you re all set to gain the claimed benefits of this diet plan, after that, use our totally free carnivore diet plan wish list.

# How To Prepare And Plan Your Carnivore Diet Meals

The complying with suggestions have aided a whole lot to stay determined and achieve my goals.

The greatest concern discovered is the objections from others, yet I have actually discovered some wonderful methods to manage them. Before we get involved in details, you can check out the food listing first if you are not familiar with it.

Currently, allow's get into it.

Know Your Why

Prior to you start with any kind of significant way of living change, it's crucial that you set out your goals.

Whether it's weight reduction, combating food allergies, or attempting to build some lean muscular tissue, you have to establish yourself a succinct goal.

Maybe it's to shed 20 lbs prior to you take place a summer trip or gain 5 lbs of lean muscular tissue in 6 months.

Whatever it is, create it down as well as publish it somewhere you can see daily.

It will certainly be a pointer to maintain you motivated.

Strategy To Commit

Sticking with a complete all-meat diet for greater than a few days or weeks takes a great deal of commitment.

The worst thing you can do is simply take it each day as well as leave it till the morning to identify what you'll be consuming.

Instead, established yourself clear objectives for the week as well as make use of the below planner as well as a shopping list to intend in advance.

I always do this on a Sunday mid-day, as well as it will certainly consist of points like how many runs and also trips to the fitness center I do, along with what I'll be eating for every dish.

You can also take a little additional time to locate new types of cuts as well as prep work approaches to add a little bit of extra variety.

If you're not keen on preparing your own dishes, you can make the most of meat shipment solutions. ButcherBox, for instance, permits you to select from their prepped-for-you meat mixes or produce your very own box as well as have it supplied to you.

It's a hassle-free means to boost your carnivore diet plan, and also most notably, you obtain top quality beef, chicken, or pork.


Social Life Preparations

Social interactions used to be among my most dreaded scenarios.

If you go to a dinner event and tell them you consume a box of donuts every early morning, have lunch at McDonalds and pizza for supper, no person will slam you excessive.

Nevertheless, tell them that your diet involves just consuming meat, and also the whole table will certainly take place the strike.

As well as god forbid there's a vegan at the table, you merely won't hear the end of it.

Right here are 2 simple techniques to make use of:

First off, tell individuals you're doing it as a result of food allergic reaction problems, and you explore this diet plan to separate the underlying reasons.

Despite having this approach, you'll still obtain remarks like: "You're completely insane, as well as it's so untrustworthy." (the vegan at the table will probably have a great deal fruitier language and an extensive tirade).

In this situation, I locate the very best point that functions are to ask whether they are interested in their very own health or yours?

9 breaks of 10 this benefits me, as well as if you obtain captured sitting alongside the vegan, then try to divert the conversation onto another thing.

Dining out.

The bright side for carnivore dieters is that there are a lot of restaurants that will certainly accommodate your requirements. Steak, as well as BBQ restaurants, are most likely your best option.

All you really require to be mindful of is the method the recipes are prepared.

Stay clear of anything that has sauces or is stir-fried with vegetables.

Unfortunately, you'll more than likely have to stay clear of Chinese and Indian dining establishments as basically, and all their dishes are hefty with sauces.

OK, so you're still with us, and you have actually jotted down your objectives and set a timeline to start.

Now it's time to help you out and intend your meat consumption for every single day of the week. I'll list out a day-to-day dish strategy based on breakfast lunch and also supper, in addition to the quantities you'll require.

This is based upon a typical height and dimension individual, yet if you have severe fat burning or muscle mass gain goals, then you will certainly need to adjust these.

Also, if you find you're still hungry after consuming these portions, then enhance the quantities slowly.

# COOK 'LESS' MEAT

Cooking less meat does not suggest you have to get rid of meat. If your family wishes to see meat or poultry on the table, then serve it, yet simply offer a smaller part. Not surprisingly, you might get some comments if you just offer half a roast chicken when everybody is utilized to seeing an entire bird! Yet, there are dozens of means to cook less without it resembling less! This is not about a pitiful part or offering much less food-simply much less meat.

Below are a few instances:

- Stir-fry- Slice up half the chicken you would typically make use of as well as change with some edamame (packed with healthy protein) beans and also an abundance of vibrant veggies. Make the stir-fry look tasty, colorful, and also bountiful on the table!

- Spaghetti- Brown half the quantity of beef to mix right into the pasta sauce. Include a variety of veggies to the marinara sauce or perhaps cooked lentils, which will certainly 'look' like meat.

- Tacos- Integrate a half portion of ground beef or ground fowl with a canister of black beans in addition to your taco seasoning mix.

- Hamburgers- Try these Half Veggie Burgers from the Excellent and also Affordable cookbook that combine hamburger, lentils (or various other beans), peppers as well as flavors to please everyone on hamburger evening!

## COOKING TIPS FOR CARNIVORES

For all the hardcore carnivores around, right here are some hacks to enhance your meat cooking video game. From defrosting meat in the microwave to sautéing meats with sugar, these tips are all you'll need.

Thawing in the Microwave

If you have actually ever defrosted meat or fish in the microwave, you probably understand that the "thaw" or low power settings are your best options for making sure that the outer edges of the food don't prepare prior to the center can defrost. But below's something you could not recognize: Setting up loose pieces of meat in a single layer with thickest components or biggest items toward the exterior will likewise guarantee even more even defrosting.

Cool Tip for Meat

Stainless steel poles are often made use of in building or crafts. Yet they can likewise come in helpful in the kitchen area, also! When cooking dense meats such as whole hen legs, beef, or pork in the stove, insert a clean, stainless steel rod into the meat. It will certainly serve as a warm conductor, enabling the within the meat to prepare at the same price as the exterior. You'll never once more have the trouble of a perfectly burnished exterior, while the insides are undercooked and also bloody.

Prepare As Soon As, Consume Two times

Wish to cook as soon as and also consume twice? Following time you're preparing boneless, skinless chicken breasts, make a few extra, after that throw the prepared poultry in a freezer bag with some Caesar dressing, and also refrigerate. Tomorrow night, cozy them in the microwave, throw over salad environment-friendlies, cut a little Parmesan cheese on top, as well as supper is ready!

Meat Wonder

All meat (except body organ meat and ground beef) ought to stand at room temperature for a few mins prior to food preparation. This allows it to brown a lot more equally, cook quicker, continue to be juicier, and also stick less when frying.

Cutting

Trimming meat right into bite-sized pieces for recipes like pasta and also stir-fries is less complicated when it's half-frozen. Place fresh meat in the freezer for two hours prior to you start supper. Or, place icy meat in the microwave and cook on the defrost setup for regarding five minutes (transforming when if you do not have a turntable). Your blade will certainly slide right through!

Sauté with Sugar

Before sautéing meats, spray a tiny quantity of sugar on the surface of the meat. The sugar will certainly respond with the juices and after that caramelize, creating a much deeper browning along with a more delicious result.

A Wonderful Usage for Stale Bread

If you're broiling steaks or chops, placed a couple of slices of stagnant bread in all-time low of the broiler frying pan to take in fat drippings. This will certainly eliminate smoking cigarettes fat, and it should also minimize any risk of a grease fire.

BEEF

## MEAT COOKING TEMPS

Beef/Lamb/Pork/Poultry

Ribeye, New York Strip, T-Bone, Porter House, Top Sirloin, Round Steak, Flat Iron, Tenderloin Filet

Sear: grill or cast iron pan on medium-high heat | 2-3 minutes per side

Flank, Skirt, Flap

Sear: grill or cast iron pan on medium-high heat | 2-3 minutes per side

Slice against the grain

Petite Tender (Teres Major)

Sear: grill or cast iron pan on medium-high heat | 2-3 minutes per side


## MEAT COOKING METHODS:

- Sear: High warm (350-400 levels F) up until outside is dark golden brown.

- Roast: High heat (350-400 levels F) in no fluid for a relatively brief time.

- Braise: Reduced warmth (225-250 degrees F) in a percentage of liquid for a very long time (4-12 hrs).

- Stew: Reduced warm (225-250 levels F) in a large quantity of fluid for a lengthy quantity of time (2-4 hrs).

- Stir fry: slim sliced.


Cut against the grain.

Hanger Steak.

Get rid of the center joint.

- Sear: grill or cast iron frying pan on medium-high warm|2-3 mins per side.

Slice versus the grain.

Tri Idea Roast.

Sear (2-3 minutes): grill or cast iron frying pan on high warmth then roast at 300 levels for 8-10 mins per extra pound.

- Stew: cube, sear, then adhere to stew dish for timing|2-4 hours.

- Brief Ribs, Korean-style cut.

- Sear: grill or actors iron frying pan|2-4 mins per side.

Chuck Roast, Short Ribs, Cross Cut Shanks, Beef Cheeks.

- Braise: long chef time, reduced warmth (200-225 levels), semi-wet environment|6-10 hrs.

- Rump Roast, Sirloin Tip Roast.

- Roast: 400 levels, completely dry warmth|12 mins per extra pound.

- Stew: dice, sear, then follow stew recipe for timing|2-4 hrs.

Brisket.

- Braise: lengthy cook time, low warm (200-225 degrees), semi-wet setting|4-6 hrs.


Beef Liver.

- Sear: cast iron frying pan on medium-high warm|1-3 minutes per side.

- Beef Tongue.

- Braise: long cook time, low warm (200-225 levels), semi-wet environment|4-6 hours.

Beef Heart.

- Sear: grill or cast iron frying pan|2-3 mins per side.

Beef Ribs.

- Braise: lengthy cook time, low heat (200-225 levels), semi-wet atmosphere|6-10 hours.

- Beef Marrow Bones.

- Roast: 400 degrees, completely dry heat|15-20 mins.

Chuck Steak.

- Sear: grill or cast iron frying pan|2-3 minutes per side.


# PORK.

Pork Rib Chops - 1 inch thick.

- Sear: grill or actors iron frying pan|2-3 minutes per side.

Sirloin Chops - 1 inch thick.

- Sear: grill or cast iron pan|2-3 mins pcr side.

- Stew: cube, sear, comply with stew dish|2-4 hours.

- Mix Fry: cut slim as well as saute above warm.

Tenderloin.

- Sear: grill or actors iron pan (2-3 mins per side), then roast at 350 degrees for 8-15 minutes.

- Stir Fry: cut thin and also saute on high warmth.

- Loin Roast (Boneless or Bone-In).

- Roast: 350 levels, dry, warm|8-10 minutes per extra pound.

Shoulder, Butt, Jowl.

- Braise: long chef time, reduced heat (200-225 levels), semi-wet environment|6-10 hours.

Infant Back Ribs, Spare Ribs.

- Braise: long cook time, low heat (200-225 degrees), semi-wet atmosphere|4-6 hours.


Pork Tummy.

- Braise: long cook time, reduced heat (200-225 levels), semi-wet environment; finish under griddle|4-6 hours.

Liver.

- Sear: grill or cast iron frying pan|2-3 minutes per side.

LAMB.

Shelf.

- Sear: grill or cast iron frying pan (4-5 minutes per side), then roast at 350 levels (8-12 mins).

Loin Chops.

- Sear: grill or actors iron pan|4-5 mins per side.

Shoulder Chops.

- Sear: grill or cast iron pan|4-5 minutes per side.

- Braise: long cook time, low heat (200-225 levels), semi-wet environment|4-6 hours.

- Stew: cube, sear, adhere to stew dish|2-4 hrs.

Leg Roast.

- Roast: 350 degrees, dry, warm|12-15 mins per pound.

Shanks, Neck Roast.

- Braise: long chef time, reduced warmth (200-225 degrees), semi-wet setting|6-10 hours.

- Stew: dice, sear, comply with stew recipe|4-6 hrs.

Liver.

- Sear: grill or actors iron pan|2-3 minutes per side.

Kidney.

- Sear: grill or cast iron pan|2-3 mins per side.

## CARNIVORE DIET RECIPE COOKBOOKS

The Carnivore Cookbook is a collection of essential recipes for the Carnivore,Keto, and Low-carb diets.

Whether you've been cooking meat for years or are just getting acquainted with your kitchen area, there's always space to find out something new and also a great cookbook can offer a deep dive into particular meat-eating subjects, from curing pork to transforming your home grill right into an Oriental barbecue. If you're aiming to increase your meaningful understanding, have a look at these recipe books that will transform any kind of residence cook right into an expert.

These publications provide you a raw structure of knowledge you'll need to recognize when on this diet. Let's start the checklist.

THE CARNIVORE DIET by Shawn Baker, MD

This is Shawns Bakers' new book. He's probably the most popular advocate for the carnivore diet. HE was on Joe Rogan's podcast, which he got a lot of attention for, as he should. He was one of the first people I heard about talk about the diet.

His book "The Carnivore Diet" is the book to get if you need to know anything about the meat-eating diet plan.

THE BIG FAT SURPRISE: WHY BUTTER, MEAT, AND CHEESE BELONG IN A HEALTHY DIET by Nina Teicholz

The fat book. This is the first book on the list I would recommend you read. One of the biggest myths about food in today's society is that "fat is bad."

The reality is that it's the exact opposite. Saturated Fat is what makes us healthy. It's what makes us burn fat for fuel instead of carbs. If you want to lose weight, eat fat

This book will open your eyes from the closed-eyelid view the modern world seduces you into.

THE MEAT EATER FISH AND GAME COOKBOOK: RECIPES AND TECHNIQUES FOR EVERY HUNTER AND ANGLER by Steven Rinella

The Meat Eater Game Guide is a must-have for all hunters and anglers. Many of us carnivores are either hunting or fishing for wild game meat. This is the ultimate cookbook for wild game.

The book guides you through how to dress big game and small game animals right after killing. Then it shows you how to cook the meat.

WEBER'S ULTIMATE GRILLING BY Weber

If you're looking for a step-by-step guide for grilling practically any recipe, look no further than Weber's Ultimate Grilling. Fired up and broiled with 125 recipes.

PROJECT SMOKE by Steven Raichlen

Project Smoke is a must-read for the barbecue meat-eater. It's a masterful work of art in the barbecue world. Project Smoke is a complete step by step guide on mastering the art of smoking meat. It's jam-packed with over 100 recipes to fulfill your every barbecue desire.

THE BRISKET CHRONICLES by Steven Raichlen

The Brisket Chronicles is your guide on how to cure, cut, braise, and smoke the world's most epic cut of meat, the brisket.

THE GAME CHEF by Angelo

The Game Chef is a bible of sorts for wild game meat-eaters. This is the best kind of meat, by the way.

ALL WILD, ALL NATURAL.

Packed with over 300 recipes of wild game, this is a must-have cookbook. If your choice of meat cuts is that of wild game, it's a no-brainer. Cooking wild game meat is slightly different than cooking meat that's packaged and sitting in a cold section in the supermarket.

GRILLING AND CAMPFIRE COOKING (EVERYDAY COOKBOOK) by Gooseberry Patch

As wild game meat-eaters, camping and grilling are the primary method and locations for our meals. Knowing how to work the grill is mandatory. Heck, I've yet to meet a carnivore that wasn't a master griller. This book shows you how to grill outside and cook with a campfire. Ideal for campers and hunters.

HUNTING, BUTCHERING, AND COOKING WILD GAME by STEVEN RINELLA

This is a dense book. When I say "book," I really mean "books." This is the first book of a two-part series.

91

The first volume is the Big Game, and the second volume is the Small Game.

## HUNTING, BUTCHERING AND COOKING WILD GAME VOLUME 2: by STEVEN RINELLA

And here is Volume 2. Just like volume 1, it is a must-have book.

## SMOKING MEAT by WILL

Get all the tools you need to smoke any cut of meat perfectly. Learn all the techniques that will help refine and make your redneck friends jealous that they don't practice smoking every day.

## MEAT EATER: ADVENTURES FROM THE LIFE OF AN AMERICAN HUNTER BY STEVEN RINELLA

Another one by Steven Rinella. He has a lot to teach and offer to our community about hunting and eating wild game meat.

## COOK'S ILLUSTRATED MEAT BOOK

The Cook's Illustrated Meat Book is packed with 425 recipes for meat and poultry that will turn you into an expert on the subject. It starts with a 27-page master class that covers shopping, storage, and seasoning (think marinating, salting, and brining) that will arm you with the necessary knowledge to ace every recipe in the book. Once inside, you'll learn techniques, offered with step-by-step illustrations, for such skills as slicing a chicken breast into cutlets, breaking down a whole bird, and carving a prime rib.

THE COMPLETE MEAT COOKBOOK by BRUCE AIDELLS AND DENNIS KELLY

The past years have introduced a meat renaissance in the USA. Gone are the days when shrink-wrapped food store meat was the only point offered. Currently, when you surf the aisles or browse the butcher counter, words like "grass-fed," "pastured," and also "organic" are the standard. Yet all of these labels can be overwhelming, which is specifically what Bruce Aidells deals with The Full Meat Cookbook.

CHARCUTERIE: THE CRAFT OF SALTING, SMOKING, AND CURING by MICHAEL RUHLMAN

There's a phase devoted to pâtés as well as terrines with recipes like English Pork Pie as well as Venison Terrine with Dried Cherries. You'll also find recipes for non-meat preservations like pickles, sauerkraut, as well as spicy smoked almonds.

FRANKLIN BARBECUE: A MEAT SMOKING MANIFESTO

93

The book then covers topics like smoke, seasoning, wood, fire, meat, and all the other essentials to great barbecue. Most of the recipes in the book are what they use at the restaurant that draws 4 or 5-hour waits on some days.

No other book has given me the same love for barbecue. Read this book, learn the techniques and understand the foundational elements of barbecue, and you will definitely start turning out some quality briskets and pork butts.

## MEATHEAD: THE SCIENCE OF GREAT BARBECUE AND GRILLING

Meathead, from AmazingRibs.com fame, is one of my favorite meat and barbecue writers or "personalities." Rather than just throw together some recipes, Meathead goes deep into the science of cooking meat. Should you really rest a steak? What causes the "stall" when smoking a pork butt? Do you need to put salt in your rubs? All these questions are answered along with hundreds more in this book. Everything in this book is tested and tested some more as well

## COOL SMOKE: THE ART OF GREAT BARBECUE

Tuffy Stone is one of the winners in competition barbecue cooks in the world, but he got his start as a classically trained chef. The book starts out with some general barbecue techniques and information but then shifts into some recipes including the ones he uses in competition

## HARDCORE CARNIVORE: COOK MEAT LIKE YOU MEAN IT

Jess Pryles is an Australian turned Texan. She was once intimidated standing at the meat counter so she took it upon herself to learn more and is now one of the top experts in the country on how to cook meat. This book reflects that knowledge and starts out with some basics every meat lover needs to know. She then delves into some great recipes. Again, they range from pretty basic to somewhat complex, but nothing that would overwhelm you.

## MEAT: EVERYTHING YOU NEED TO KNOW

There are probably very few people in this country that have handled more meat than Pat LaFrieda. Pat and his family run a huge butcher operation in NYC and supply meat to many of the top restaurants in the city and across the country.

## NOTE

The Carnivore Cookbook explores what our bodies were actually developed to absorb and gives compelling proof that we were designed to be primarily meat-eaters. In this book, you will learn why all plants included a drawback. Antinutrients are chemicals and also compounds that act as all-natural chemicals or supports for the plants versus being consumed. Maria discusses how antinutrients can burglarize your body of minerals and also other nutrients and lead to autoimmune issues and also dripping intestine. Consists of more than 100 tasty meat-focussed recipes, carnivore meal plans, and grocery store list to make the diet plan easy to follow.

## THE BEST CARNIVORE RECIPES

Does a meat-only diet plan appear fascinating to you? If you enjoy a good steak (and also meats, in general), a carnivore diet plan might just be the tastiest diet plan you'll ever attempt. Nonetheless, initially, it may seem a bit tough to prepare meals that include only meats.

This collection includes every one of my favored meaty recipes-- and also you don't require to be a cook to prepare these! They are best when you yearn for a passionate dinner or when you don't take place to have fresh veggies available.

Smokey Bacon Meatballs

Ingredients: chicken breasts or ground chicken, pieces of bacon, egg, garlic, onion powder, liquid smoke, avocado, or olive oil.

Using a blend of bacon and hen with a hint of smokiness included for added flavor, these have to be several of the tastiest meatballs ever before! They simply have the ideal balance of meat and also fat to make them unctuous and juicy, yet they hold with each other actually well. These meatballs are really reduced in carbohydrates yet packed with taste as well as they even drop well with the children!


Steak au Poivre

Components: filet mignon or similar steak, salt, peppercorns, a sprig of thyme, garlic, ghee.

Steak is among those outstanding meals that are frequently served at dinner celebrations, but it can be an excellent suggestion when you are following a particular diet plan, to treat yourself to steak every so often. This is a simple dish, but the crushed peppercorns include such a unique flavor to the meat that it is worth a try! Attempt not to overcook the steak as the taste is best when the steak is medium uncommon.

Crunchy Indian Chicken Drumsticks

ACTIVE INGREDIENTS

- 10 poultry drumsticks

- 2-- 3 Tablespoons salt (it'll depend on the salt you're using).

- 3-- 4 Tbsps garam masala (include even more for extra taste) (this is the one I use).

- 1/2 Tbsp of coconut oil for oiling baking tray.

GUIDELINES.

- Preheat stove to 450F (230C).

- Grease a huge cooking tray with coconut oil.

- Mix the salt as well as the garam masala with each other in a bowl.

- Make certain the drumsticks are not also damp (or else it won't get crunchy).

- Coat each drumstick with the combination and also put on the cooking tray. Make sure the drumsticks are not touching each other on the tray.

- Bake for 40 minutes.

NUTRITION.

Offering Dimension: 5 drumsticks.


Garlic Ghee Baked Poultry Bust Recipe.

COMPONENTS.

- 1 hen bust.

- 1 teaspoon garlic powder.

- 1 Tbsp ghee (usage of coconut oil or olive oil for AIP).

- 2 cloves garlic, chopped (or 2 teaspoons additional garlic powder).

- 1 tsp of sea salt.

- 1 tsp chives, diced (optional).

DIRECTIONS.

- Preheat stove to 350F (180C).

- The area the hen bust on a piece of aluminum foil as well as position the garlic powder, ghee, chopped fresh garlic, and also sea salt over it. Scrub everything over the poultry breast.

- Fold up the aluminum foil to ensure that it covers the poultry bust. Place it on a cooking tray and cook for half an hour. The chicken breast ought to be cooked through (no pinkness in the center and your meat thermometer must read over 165F (75C) for the middle of the chicken breast).

- Cut the hen bust in half or into pieces and also spray diced chives on the top.

- Serve with more ghee as well as salt to preference.


Marinated Grilled Flank Steak.

ACTIVE INGREDIENTS.

- 3 lbs flank steak.

- 1 cup of coconut oil or olive oil.

- 2/3 cup coconut aminos.

- 1/2 cup apple cider vinegar.

- juice from 1 lemon.

- 2 tbsps of mustard.

- 6 cloves of garlic, squashed.

- 1 tbsp grated ginger (ideally fresh ginger).

- 1 tablespoon paprika.

- 1 tablespoon dried out the chopped onion or onion powder.

- 1 tablespoon salt.

- 2 tsps dried out thyme.

- 1 teaspoon chili powder.

DIRECTIONS.

- Cut the flank steak right into workable pieces if it's not already cut so.

- Develop the sauce utilizing all the components (other than the steak).

- Location each piece of steak into a ziplock bag and also divide the sauce equally between the bags.

- Seal the bags and season overnight ideally. I such as to use olive oil if seasoning overnight or melted coconut oil if only marinating for an hour at room temperature level.

- Then simply grill them! You can use a meat thermostat to obtain the steak to the rareness you want. Typically, for medium uncommon, I barbecue it on a hot grill with the cover down 3 mins on each side (internal temperature level of the grill is 500-600F).

NOTES.

Coconut oil will certainly solidify when the temperature level goes down-- I don't discover this to be bothersome if you cover the steak well with the marinade, but an option is to utilize olive oil, which functions just as well.

Bifteck Hache (French Hamburgers) Recipe.

ACTIVE INGREDIENTS.

- For the hamburgers.

- 2 Tbsps (30 ml) ghee or coconut oil, slightly thawed.

- 1 onion, carefully diced (separated into 2 portions).

- 1.5 pound (680 g) hamburger.

- 1 egg.

- 1 Tablespoon (2 g) fresh thyme leaves.

- Salt and pepper to preference.

- Added ghee or coconut oil to cook with.

- For the sauce.

- 1/2 mug (120 ml) beef stock.

- 2 Tablespoons (30 ml) additional ghee.

- 1/4 cup (8 g) parsley, finely sliced.

DIRECTIONS.

- The area the 2 Tablespoons of ghee or coconut oil into a frying pan as well as chef half the diced onions in the pan up until they turn transparent.

- Allow the onions cool down and then add them (including the oil in the frying pan) to a mixing bowl with the ground beef, egg, thyme leaves, salt, as well as pepper.

- Mix well as well as create 6-8 patties from the meat mixture.

- Cook the patties in a frying pan with additional ghee or coconut oil until both sides are well browned (make flatter patties if you like the burgers to be well-done).

- For the sauce, put out the remaining oil from the frying pan, include the 2 Tablespoons of extra ghee as well as saute the remainder of the diced onions. Then add in the beef stock as well as reduce the sauce down for a couple of mins. Add in the parsley and serve the sauce with the hamburgers.

NOTES.

All dietary information is estimated and also based on per offering quantities.

NOURISHMENT.

Serving Dimension: 2 Burgers Calories: 460 Sugar: 0 g Fat: 36 g Carbohydrates: 1 g Fiber: 0 g Healthy protein: 35 g.

Grilled Chicken Drumsticks with Garlic Marinate.

This is a straightforward smoked meal-- best now that the climate is warmer and also the grill can be terminated up once again!

ACTIVE INGREDIENTS.

- 10 chicken drumsticks.

- 1 1/2 cups of olive oil.

- 1 head of garlic (around 10 cloves).

- juice from 1 lemon.

- 1 tbsp of sea salt.

- 1/2 teaspoon of pepper.

GUIDELINES.

- Place the olive oil, garlic, lemon juice, sea salt, as well as pepper right into a mixer or food mill as well as puree. This is the marinade.

- Rub the hen drumsticks in the marinade. After that position, the hen with the sauce right into Ziploc bags and also placed in the refrigerator. Sauce for a minimum of 2 hrs.

- Grill the chicken drumsticks.

NOTES.

All nutritional data are estimated and based upon per offering quantities.

NUTRITION.

Offering Dimension: 2-3 hen drumsticks Calories: 660 Sugar: 0 Fat: 56 g Carbohydrates: 4 g Fiber: 0 Healthy protein: 36 g.


Grilled Cumin Crusted Lamb Chops Recipe.

Make the cumin mixture with cumin, paprika, chili powder, and also salt. Mix it together well-- taste a little bit to see to it it's the appropriate mix for your preferences (add even more salt or chili powder as required).

105

SUMMARY.

Makes around 20 lamb chops.

COMPONENTS.

- 2 lambs ribs (3 pounds).

- 3/4 cup cumin powder.

- 3 Tablespoons paprika.

- 1 tsp chili powder (more if preferred).

- 1 Tbsp salt (less if preferred).

GUIDELINES.

- Cut the lambs ribs into private lamb chops.

- Combine the cumin powder, paprika, chili powder, and also salt.

- Dip each lamb slice into the blend.

- Beginning the grill and place on the most affordable temperature.

- Place the lamb chops on the grill and also cook for 5 mins with the cover down. Don't allow the temperature inside the grill to go above 350F.

- After that, turn the lamb chops every 2-3 mins till done to the level you delight in.

Garlic Bacon Covered Poultry Bites Recipe.

INGREDIENTS.

- 1 huge hen breast, cut into little attacks (approx 22--27 pieces).

- 8-- 9 thin pieces of bacon, reduced right into thirds.

- 3 Tbsps garlic powder (or 6 crushed garlic if chosen).

GUIDELINES.

Preheat oven to 400F (205C) as well as line a baking tray with aluminum foil.

- The area the garlic powder into a dish as well as dip each chicken bite right into the garlic powder.

- Wrap each short bacon piece around each garlic chicken bite. Place the bacon-wrapped poultry attacks on the cooking tray. Try to space them out so they're not touching.

- Bake for 25-30 minutes till the bacon turns crispy. Turn the pieces after 15 minutes if you can bear in mind.

NOTES.

All nutritional data are approximated as well as based upon per serving amounts.

NOURISHMENT.

Calories: 230 Sugar: 2 g Fat: 13 g Carbs: 5 g Fiber: 1 g Healthy protein: 22 g.


Garlic Ghee Pan-Fried Cod Recipe.

COMPONENTS.

- 4 cod filets (approx 0.3 lb each).

- 3 Tablespoons ghee.

- 6 cloves of garlic, minced.

- 1 Tablespoon garlic powder (optional).

- Salt to taste.

DIRECTIONS.

- Thaw the ghee in a frying pan.

- Add in half the minced garlic to the pan.

- The area the cod filets right into the pan as well as a chef on medium to high warmth. Sprinkle with salt as well as garlic powder.

- As the fish chefs, it'll transform from translucent to a strong white shade. Await the white shade to creep half-way up the side of the fish and then flip the fish and also include the remainder of the minced garlic.

- Prepare up until the whole filet turns a solid white shade (it must likewise flake easily).

- Serve with several of the garlic and ghee from the frying pan.

NOTES.

All dietary information is approximated and also based on per offering amounts.

NOURISHMENT.

Calories: 160 Sugar: 0 g Fat: 7 g Carbohydrates: 1 g Fiber: 0 g Healthy protein: 21 g.

High end-- Vapor Your Own Lobster

COMPONENTS

- 4 lobster tails (approx. 1 lb with shell).

- Tools-- a steamer.

- seasoning/ghee (optional-- I like my lobster level).

DIRECTIONS.

- Thaw the lobster tails if they're frozen.

- Fill up the pot halfway with water. Location the steamer accessory on top of the pot and placed the cover on top of the steamer accessory. Currently, warm the pot on high warmth until the water is boiling.

- After the water is steaming, very carefully place the lobster tails (preferably with tongs, so you don't melt yourself) onto the cleaner add-on-- keep in mind to place the cover back on.

- Set a timer for specifically 10 mins, and get rid of the lobster tails immediately when the timer goes off. If you're making use of fresh lobster, you can heavy steam it for 8-9 mins. Note that the moment adjustments depending on just how much lobster you're steaming! Check the blog post for even more timing choices.

NUTRITION.

Serving Size: 1 lobster tail.


Poultry, as well as Bacon Sausages Recipe.

These poultry bacon sausages are tasty as well as easy and fast to make. And also, they fit the Paleo,

Ketogenic, and also AIP (Paleo autoimmune method) diet plans. Simply omit the egg if you're allergic to eggs or if you get on AIP. If you're ok eating eggs, then I highly recommend including it in as it makes the sausages moister.

ACTIVE INGREDIENTS.

- 2 large poultry busts, or usage 1 lb ground chicken.

- 2 slices bacon, cooked, and also gotten into smidgens.

- 1 egg, whisked (leave out for AIP).

- 2 Tablespoons Italian flavoring.

- 2 tsps garlic powder.

- 2 tsps onion powder.

- Salt and also pepper.

DIRECTIONS.

- Preheat stove to 425 F (220 C).

- Food procedure all the components together.

- Kind 12 thin patties (1/2-inch thick) from the meat blend and also position on a baking tray lined with aluminum foil (so you do not need to wash the cooking tray).

- Bake for 20 mins. Get in touch with a meat thermostat that the inner temperature of a patty near the middle of the tray is 170 F (76 C).

- Trendy and also store in the fridge or fridge freezer (reheat them conveniently in the early mornings in the skillet or in the microwave).

-( You can likewise pan-fry the raw sausages instead of putting them into the stove.).

NOTES.

All nutritional information is approximated and based upon per offering quantities.

NOURISHMENT.

Calories: 370 Sugar: 1 g Fat: 21 g Carbohydrates: 3 g Fiber: 1 g Healthy protein: 40 g.


Exactly how To Boil A Dungeness Crab.

COMPONENTS.

- 1 Dungeness crab.

INSTRUCTIONS.

- Place the crab into a large pot of cool water-- use lengthy tongs for real-time crabs.

- Bring the pot of cold water to the boil slowly.

- Boil for 7-8 mins per pound of crab.


Pan-Fried Tilapia Meal.

PAN-FRIED TILAPIA Season the tilapia fillet with some salt. The area the filets into a frying pan with coconut oil on a tool warmth. Let the filets prepare up until the majority of the tilapia modifications color (turns from opaque to white). Make use of a broad spatula to turn the filets over gently. Prepare for a few even more mins and also offer.

ACTIVE INGREDIENTS.

- 2 cups carrots, peeled.

- 2 tbsps coconut milk.

- GUIDELINES.

- Steam the carrots till they're tender.

- Puree the carrots in a mixer with the 2 tbsps of coconut milk.


Paleo Baked Rosemary Salmon Dish.

The olive oil and also the foil (or parchment paper) help to keep the salmon moist also if you happen to overcook it! So you truly can not go wrong with this very easy Paleo dish no matter how poor of a cook you assume you are.

SUMMARY.

Obtain this Paleo baked rosemary salmon dish below. It's very easy and also deliciously moist. Plus, this recipe is Keto as well as AIP-friendly.

INGREDIENTS.

- 2 salmon fillets (fresh or defrosted).

- 1 tablespoon fresh rosemary leaves.

- 1/4 mug (4 tbsps) olive oil.

- 1 tsp salt (optional or to preference).

GUIDELINES.

- Preheat the oven to 350F (175C).

- Mix the olive oil, rosemary, as well as salt together in a bowl.

- Massage the mix onto the salmon fillets.

- Cover each fillet in an item of aluminum foil with a few of the remaining blend.

- Bake for 25-30 minutes.

NUTRITION.

Serving Size: salmon fillet.

Pan-Fried Pork Tenderloin.

This meal calls for zero preparation and also uses very extremely couple of active ingredients. So, exactly how do you cook scrumptious pork in a frying pan?

INGREDIENTS.

- 1 lb pork tenderloin.

- salt as well as pepper to taste.

- 1 tbsp coconut oil.

GUIDELINES.

- Cut the 1 lb pork tenderloin in fifty percent (to produce 2 equal shorter fifty percent).

- Place the 1 tablespoon of coconut oil into a frying pan on medium heat.

- After the coconut oil thaws, place the 2 pork tenderloin items into the pan.

- Leave the pork to prepare on its side. As soon as that side is prepared, transform making use of tongs to cook the other sides. Keep turning and also preparing up until the pork looks prepared on all sides.

- Cook all sides of the pork till the meat thermometer shows an interior temperature level of just listed below 145F (63C). The pork will go on cooking a bit after you take it out of the frying pan.

- Allow the pork sit for a few mins and after that slice into 1-inch thick slices with a sharp knife.

NOTES.

All dietary data are approximated as well as based on per offering quantities.

NOURISHMENT.

Calories: 330 Sugar: 0 g Fat: 15 g Carbs: 0 g Fiber: 0 g Healthy protein: 47 g.


Spicy Paleo Dry Rub Ribs.

The rub is an easy combination of salt, paprika, garlic powder, and onion powder. They're all components you can easily buy at your local supermarket in the US.

COMPONENTS.

- 2-pound pork spare ribs.

- 1 Tablespoon salt.

- 2 Tbsps paprika.

- 1 Tablespoon garlic powder.

- 1 Tablespoon onion powder.

- 1/2 teaspoon chili powder or cayenne pepper (optional).

INSTRUCTIONS.

- Cut the ribs to make sure that they remain in slabs of approx. 4 ribs.

- Location the ribs in a pot of water (make sure the ribs are submerged in the water) and also steam for 1 hr. [Optional] Make use of a spoon to remove any type of residue drifting in the water.

- Preheat stove to 325F.

- Mix with each other the salt, paprika, garlic powder, onion powder, as well as chili pepper to develop the rub. Preference the rub to see if you choose more of one seasoning.

- The area the boiled ribs in a baking frying pan as well as dip each collection of ribs into the rub. Location foil over the baking pan and also bake for 40 mins. Eliminate the foil as well as cook for another 20 mins.

- Add more salt to preference (optional).

NOURISHMENT.

Offering Dimension: 6-8 ribs.


Slow Cooker Pork.

All you need is some pork shoulder (this is a 2-pound pork shoulder collar I obtained from my butchers). After that, I included a couple of spices to it (ginger powder, salt, Szechuan peppercorns) and a few prunes. DO NOT ADD ANY LIQUID!

INGREDIENTS.

- 2 lb pork shoulder (or pork shoulder collar).

- 1 tbsp salt (or to taste).

- 1 tbsp ginger powder.

- 1 tablespoon Szechuan peppercorns.

- 4 prunes (optional).

DIRECTIONS.

- Place the pork into the slow stove (do not reduce up).

- Sprinkle the spices onto the meat.

- Include the prunes.

- Establish a slow-moving cooker for 8 hours on low warmth setup.

- Transform meat over after 6 hrs; however, do not rive meat.

NOTES.

All dietary data are approximated and also based upon per serving quantities.

NUTRITION.

Serving Dimension: 1/2 pound Calories: 422 Fat: 28 g Protein: 40 g.


Slow Stove Paleo Jerk Chicken.

The word "jerk" stems from Spanish words indicating dried out meat (thus the food beef jerky). So jerk poultry, which is a popular meal in Jamaica (see image below), is made with a spicy, completely dry rub.

Although this dish is generally grilled, it's in fact, much easier in the slow-moving cooker! Just massage the flavors on the chicken and cook away.

INGREDIENTS.

- 5 drumsticks and also 5 wings (or you can use a whole chicken or 5 chicken breasts).

- 4 teaspoons of salt.

- 4 teaspoons of paprika.

- 1 teaspoon of cayenne pepper.

- 2 teaspoons of onion powder.

- 2 tsps of thyme.

- 2 teaspoons of white pepper.

- 2 tsps of garlic powder.

- 1 tsps of black pepper.

INSTRUCTIONS.

- Mix all the flavors together in a dish to make a rub for the poultry. If you don't desire your hen to be hot, after that, omit the chili pepper as well as instead add in even more onion powder, yet keep in mind that the paprika will certainly still make it slightly spicy.

- Laundry the chicken meat in cool water briefly. Place the cleaned hen meat right into the dish with a snag, as well as massage the flavors onto the meat thoroughly-- try to get it under the hen skin if you can. The wings and drumsticks function well here due to the fact that you can rub the spices under the skin quickly.

- Area each piece of hen covered with the spices right into the sluggish stove (no liquid required).

- Establish the slow-cooker on medium or low warm (325F if your sluggish stove has a temperature level controller), and chef for 5-6 hours or until the hen meat falls off the bone (slow stove times can vary substantially).

- You can offer the chicken with the bone on or take the bones out, considering that the meat diminishes so quickly.

NOURISHMENT.

Offering Size: 2-3 items of the hen.


Lemon Ghee Roast Poultry Dish.

Lemon chicken differs extremely worldwide. This lemon ghee roast hen dish adds just the right amount of flavor to the juicy poultry.

Lemon Poultry All Over The World.

While this paleo tackle lemon chicken is baked, many countries all over the world deep-fry lemon chicken.

•        In Canada, a Chinese-food design variation of lemon poultry is deep-fried as well as covered with a sweet lemon sauce. In a similar way, in Australia and also New Zealand, they coat the poultry in batter, fry it, as well as for drizzle lemon sauce over the meal.

•        In France, you may come across lemon chicken prepared with Dijon mustard. Over in Italy, you begin getting closer to this recipe. There, the lemon hen is a whole baked chicken cooked in Gewurztraminer, thyme, and lemon juice.

•        In America, Italian lemon poultry is usually prepared with capers.

•        INGREDIENTS

•        - 1 entire hen (4 pounds or 2 Kg) eliminate giblets

•        - 1 lemon, zested and also sliced

•        - 1 lemon, halved

•        - 1/2 cup (120 ml) ghee

•        - Salt.

- INSTRUCTIONS.

- - Preheat oven to 350 F (175 C).

- - Combine salt and also lemon passion and scrub all over the poultry.

- - Salt the inside of the poultry as well as stuff the 2 lemon halves inside along with 1/4 mug of ghee.

- - Massage the remainder of the ghee outside of the chicken.

- - The area into a toasting frying pan. The area the lemon pieces around the poultry in the pan.

- - Roast for 105 minutes. Get in touch with a meat thermostat to make certain the interior temperature level of the poultry meat is 165 F (74 C).

- - If your hen is larger or smaller sized, you will certainly require to change the cooking time.

- - Get rid of the frying pan from the oven, as well as put up a lightweight aluminum tent around the frying pan to keep the warmth and juices in. Relax the poultry for around 10 mins. After that slice and also appreciate it!

- NOTES.

•       All dietary information is estimated and also based upon per serving quantities.

•       NUTRITION.

•       Calories: 432 Sugar: 0 g Fat: 30 g Carbs: 0 g Fiber: 0 g Protein: 43 g.

•

•       AIP Italian Burgers Recipe.

•       Grass-fed beef burgers are not just AIP, Paleo, as well as Keto, but they're likewise simply truly delicious and easy to make.

•       So, whip these up whatever diet plan you get on. You can likewise switch out the spices or include some vegetables to change the tastes.

•       Below are some different seasoning options for AIP burgers.

•       - Thai Burgers-- Chopped fresh basil leaves with a dash of coconut aminos.

•       - Onion Burgers-- Carefully chopped environment-friendly onions with onion powder.

•       - Garlic Burgers-- Carefully cut onions with garlic powder.

- - Veggie Burgers-- Carefully chopped asparagus, spinach, as well as eco-friendly onions.

- Evaluate them out as well as see which one is your fave. Personally, I find the onions with garlic are delicious every time!

- ACTIVE INGREDIENTS.

- - 1 pound of grass-fed hamburger (450 g).

- - 2 Tbsps of Italian seasoning (6 g).

- - 2 Tablespoons of garlic powder (20 g).

- - 1 Tbsp of onion powder (7 g).

- GUIDELINES.

- - Mix all the active ingredients with each other well and also develop hamburger patties from the mix.

- - Grill or pan-fry in coconut oil up until done to your preference.

- NOTES.

- All nutritional data are estimated and based on per offering quantities.

- NOURISHMENT.

- Calories: 640 Sugar: 3 g Fat: 48 g Carbohydrates: 9 g Fiber: 1 g Healthy protein: 39 g.

- 

- AIP Bacon-Wrapped Salmon Dish.

- This AIP bacon-wrapped salmon recipe is a suit made in heaven. It's a luxurious low-carb day-night sort of meal you can make fast.

- ACTIVE INGREDIENTS.

- - 2 filets of salmon, fresh or icy (340 g).

- - 4 slices of bacon (112 g).

- - 1 Tbsp of olive oil (15 ml).

- - 2 Tbsps of tarragon (32 g), to garnish.

- - Lemon wedges, to serve.

- GUIDELINES.

- Preheat the stove to 350 ° F( 180 ° C). - Rub the salmon fillets completely dry. Cover bacon around the fillets.

- - Place fillets onto a toasting tray and drizzle with the olive oil. Bake for 15-20 mins.

- - Serve garnished with sliced tarragon as well as lemon wedges.

- NOTES.

- All nutritional data are approximated as well as based on per serving quantities.

- NUTRITION.

- Calories: 776 Sugar: 0 g Fat: 63 g Carbohydrates: 0 g Fiber: 0 g Protein: 48 g.

- 

- 3-Ingredient Crispy Hen Thighs Dish.

- Do not think that hen can be juicy and tasty if it hasn't been fried or breaded? I invite you to taste for yourself simply exactly how scrumptious this keto hen upper legs dish can be without turning to a deep fryer.

- Baked vs. Fried.

- Sure, deep-fried foods can taste good. But their flavor originates from swimming in fat, which can work against your efforts to be healthy. Fat can be good, however too much fat can work against your weight-loss objectives.

- Fried foods include a lot of calories contrasted to their baked counterparts. Constant usage of fried meat is additionally related to an increased threat of colon, pancreatic, and also prostate cancer.

- Luckily, this 3-ingredient crispy keto hen thighs dish will certainly offer you poultry that tastes so

127

excellent you will not wish for the fried variation. And you will miss some possible pitfalls for your health.

- COMPONENTS.

- - 12 hen thighs (with the skin on).

- - 4 Tablespoons of olive oil (60 ml) or avocado oil.

- - 2 Tablespoons salt (30 g).

- - INSTRUCTIONS.

- - Preheat stove to 450F (230C).

- - Rub salt on each hen upper leg in the combination and also put on a greased cooking tray. Make sure the upper legs are not touching each various other on the tray. Drizzle the olive oil or avocado oil over the upper poultry legs.

- - Bake for 40 minutes until the skin is crunchy.

- NOTES.

- All dietary information is estimated and also based on per serving amounts.

- Internet Carbohydrates: 0 g.

- NOURISHMENT.

- Calories: 713 Sugar: 0 g Fat: 56 g Carbohydrates: 0 g Fiber: 0 g Healthy protein: 48 g.

-

- Three Ingredient Steak Sauté Dish.

- Making steak does not need to be a labor and also time-intensive procedure. This very easy three-ingredient keto steak sauté dish is best for a hectic weeknight. You simply require steak, onions, as well as garlic.

- Buying the Best Ribeye.

- The success or failure of your steak is often established at the supermarket. While there are a lot of ways to mess up a steak in your home, by and large, the largest consider just how scrumptious (or otherwise) your steak originates from your selection at the supermarket, farmer's market, butcher, or anywhere you acquire your meat.

- ACTIVE INGREDIENTS.

- - 1 beef ribeye steak, cut.

- - 1/2 onion, peeled off, and also sliced.

- - 2 cloves of garlic, diced.

- - 2 Tbsps (30 ml) avocado oil to cook with.

- DIRECTIONS.

- - Include avocado oil to a frying pan and sauté the steak, onion, and garlic.

- NOTES.

- All nutritional information is approximated and based on per serving amounts.

- Internet Carbohydrates: 6 g.

- NOURISHMENT.

- Calories: 798 Sugar: 3 g Fat: 70 g Carbohydrates: 7 g Fiber: 1 g Healthy protein: 35 g.

- 

- Lemon Chicken Recipe.

- This lemon chicken recipe is so quick and easy you can make it after work. Grab a bundle of cauliflower rice (yes, that's a thing now!) and also, you're all set for the best dish!

- Different Cuts of Chicken.

- Just how typically do you pass the fowl in the grocery store in a zombie-like state, just to get the hen breast by habit?

• There are various other gamers in the hen game, you recognize. This specific recipe asks for either chicken upper legs or drumsticks. Allow's speak about those.

• Hen Thighs.

• The meat on thighs is darker as well as firmer than hen busts. Most individuals consider it to be more delicious too.

• It's a good idea to maintain the skin on when you prepare thighs. This aids the meat to continue to be tender and also juicy.

• Drumsticks.

• Children and also the young in mind seem to enjoy feasting on drumsticks, which frequently plead to be eaten by hand.

• A popular barbeque alternative, they begin the bone. They're affordable and also very easy to collaborate with. Once again, I would certainly guidance maintaining the skin on when dealing with drumsticks.

ACTIVE INGREDIENTS.

• Tbsps (30ml) olive oil for the marinade.

• hen thighs or drumsticks (with the skin on).

- 2 Tablespoons thyme leaves.

- 2 Tbsps (30 ml) lemon juice.

- Salt and freshly ground black pepper.

- 2 Tablespoons (30 ml) olive oil, to prepare with.

- 2 cloves garlic, peeled off as well as diced.

- 1 lemon, sliced up.

INSTRUCTIONS.

- Preheat stove to 350 F (180 C).

- Mix the 2 Tablespoons of olive oil, thyme, lemon juice, salt, as well as pepper together in a bowl and scrub the blend on the chicken items, making certain to scrub under the skin.

- Add the other 2 Tablespoons of olive oil to a big fry pan on high warm and also area the chicken pieces right into the warm frying pan skin-side down. Fry till the skin is crispy. Turn the poultry items over and also prepare the opposite for a few mins.

- Transfer the chicken to a baking tray, gather any leftover sauce along with the lemon slices and also garlic — Cook for 20 mins (examine the poultry is totally prepared).

• Offer garnished with a scattering of fresh thyme leaves as well as an offer over prepared cauliflower rice.

NOTES.

• All dietary information is approximated and based upon per offering amounts.

• Internet Carbohydrates: 1 g.

NOURISHMENT.

• Calories: 638 Sugar: 0 g Fat: 56 g Carbs: 1 g Fiber: 0 g Healthy protein: 32 g.

•


Crockpot Shredded Poultry.

If you're looking for the excellent canvas for a healthy as well as low-carb lunch or dinner, look no more than this Keto crockpot shredded poultry! It could not be much easier to make, as well as only needs 5 mins of hands-on time. Make a batch on a careless Sunday mid-day and also enjoy juicy, tasty hen all week long.

SUMMARY.

• This easy crockpot dish will come to be a staple in your residence.

COMPONENTS.

- 4 chicken busts.

- 1 cup (240 ml) poultry broth.

- 4 cloves garlic.

- 1/2 onion, cut.

- Salt and pepper, to taste.

- 1 Tablespoon Italian seasoning.

GUIDELINES.

- Include whatever to the crockpot.

- Cook on reduced for 6 hours.

- Shred the meat with your forks.

- Enjoy instantly in numerous meals (e.g., salads, lettuce wraps, sautes, or soups) or freeze in private packs for future use.

- Enjoy with guacamole or on top of a salad with Caesar's clothing.

- NOTES.

- All dietary data are estimated as well as based on per offering quantities.

- Web Carbs: 1 g.

NOURISHMENT.

- Calories: 201 Sugar: 0 g Fat: 10 g Carbohydrates: 1 g Fiber: 0 g Healthy protein: 24 g.

- Body organ Meats.

-

Rosemary Liver Hamburgers.

The liver is so great for us. However, the taste even obtains me sometimes! So I slip them into things, and also burgers are excellent candidates. After that, you add some great spices to cover it up a lot more. Of course, if you love the preference of liver, then there's no requirement to do any of this!

COMPONENTS.

- 2 lbs ground grass-fed beef.

- 1 lb ground liver (you can food process your liver and then drain pipes the excess blood).

- 1/4-- 1/2 cup rosemary, carefully sliced.

- 1 tbsp chili pepper flakes (less if you don't desire it as well spicy).

- 2 tablespoons oregano.

- 1 tsp black pepper.

GUIDELINES.

Mix all the active ingredients together well.

 Kind thin burger patties with your hands.

• 	Grill the burgers until completely cooked with.


Baked Bone Marrow Dish.

Are you prepared for some pure decadence? It does not get a lot more polished than this. Baked bone marrow is one of the supreme recipes that are spent lavishly on at elegant five-star dining establishments. As opposed to investing an arm and also a leg on a couple of bites of richness, making this meal in the house is much simpler than one would anticipate. The various other terrific components about bone marrow are that it can collaborate with your carnivore diet plan. This baked bone marrow recipe will certainly not only reveal you what an amazing cook you can be, yet it will certainly also deserve the initiative when you take that first bite.

SUMMARY.

Decadent and abundant, baked bone marrow goes well with pleasant, plump sliced tomatoes, which offer a much-needed level of acidity to puncture all that wonderful fattiness.

COMPONENTS.

- 4 bone marrow fifty percent.

- Salt and also pepper, to taste.

- 2 teaspoons (10 ml) lemon juice.

- 1/2 tomato, sliced (to offer with).

- 1 mug salad greens.

GUIDELINES.

- Preheat the oven to 350 F (175 C).

- Prepare the bones by positioning them on a foil-lined baking tray (as the fat makes when the marrow chefs).

- Bake for 20 mins (longer if the bones are thicker). The marrow will certainly be browned and a little bubbling. And some of the fat will certainly have rendered and streamed off.

- To offer, sprinkle salt and also pepper over the marrow and drizzle some lemon juice.

- Offer with tomato pieces as well as a green side salad.

NOTES.

All nutritional data are approximated and based on per offering amounts.

NUTRITION.

Calories: 440 Sugar: 0 g Fat: 48 g Carbohydrates: 1 g Fiber: 0 g Protein: 4 g.

## DELICIOUS BEEF AND LIVER BURGER RECIPE.

ACTIVE INGREDIENTS.

•       1.25 pounds Ground Beef, I choose 20% ground beef.

•       1/4 lb Poultry livers.

•       1 tsp of sea salt.

•       1 teaspoon ground black pepper, you can add even more if you would like.

•       1 1/2 tsp coriander.

•       1 teaspoon Chicken Seasoning.

•       1/2 Red tool Onion, peeled.

GUIDELINES.

•       In your food mill, include your poultry liver and red onion.

- Pulse till it's a mush.

- Next include the hamburger and also all the spices.

- Pulse the food mill for roughly 1 min till the blend is mixed.

- It will certainly be slightly sticky, so you will certainly wish to damp your hands prior to shaping the patties.

 Forming the blend into four 4" large pattie

Cook/Grill patties until it reaches your desired doneness (is that a word?).

Enjoy on a lettuce cover or burger bun.

NUTRITION INFO: RETURN: 4 OFFERING SIZE: g.

Amount Per Portion: CALORIES: 396 HYDROGENATED FAT: 11g CHOLESTEROL: 198mg SODIUM: 696mg PROTEIN: 29g.


GRILLED BEEF HEART.

Grilled Beef Heart has a taste and texture that are remarkably similar to that of a good barbequed steak or roast beef. Risk try it, wager you'll ENJOY it!

COMPONENTS.

•        1 beef heart, about 1kg|2.2 lb.

•        1/2 cup balsamic vinegar.

•        Salt and pepper to taste, be generous!

•        A fair quantity of food preparation, fat, ghee, lard, or coconut oil.

INSTRUCTIONS.

•        Wash the heart well under cool running water as well as pat it really completely dry.

•        Cut the heart open (if your butcher hasn't done that currently) and also eliminate any visible strings, arteries as well as blood vessels that might have been left behind; cut off excess fat and reserve.

•        Location the heart to marinate overnight in balsamic vinegar.

•        When you prepare to barbecue the heart, pat it truly completely dry once more, as well as spray generously with salt and pepper on both sides.

- Cut the heart in half if necessary, so it fits in your skillet (or if you intend to save some of it for another dish).

- Thaw a reasonable amount of cooking fat in a big heavy frying pan set over high heat. Grill the beef heart without moving the meat for 5-6 minutes per side, or until a good golden crust kind.

- Remove the meat to a plate, outdoor tents loosely with lightweight aluminum foil and allow it rest for 15 minutes.

- Cut fairly very finely against the grain as well as offer.

NOTES.

This is equally tasty cold. It tastes much like roast beef.

Nutrition Details.

calories: 357kcal, carbohydrates: 4g, healthy protein: 54g, fat: 12g, saturated fat: 4g, cholesterol: 375mg, salt: 301mg, potassium: 891mg, sugar: 3g, vitamin c: 6mg, calcium: 27mg, iron: 13mg.

Easy Beef Heart Steak.

Very few people like heart meat any longer, and it is a pity because, like the old Chinese saying goes: "Consume the organ you want to heal." Well, our contemporary hearts need much healing, especially in a strictly physiological feeling.

The beef heart contains all essential amino acids, zinc, selenium and also phosphorus.

It has greater than double the elastin and also collagen than other cuts of meat as well as a very focused resource of coenzyme Q10, additionally known as CoQ10.

Ingredients.

•       1 tablespoon ghee.

•       4 pieces of beef heart 1" thick.

•       2 tablespoon rosemary-infused olive oil (or simple olive oil).

•       salt and pepper to taste.

Instructions.

•       Take heart pieces from the marinade and rub dry.

•       Warmth a cast iron skillet with the ghee on a high fire for 2/3 mins.

•	Lay meat in the skillet. The temperature level ought to be high sufficient to sizzle.

•	Cook for 5 min on each side up until perfectly browned outside but still pink in the middle.

•	Drizzle with the rosemary instilled olive oil.

•	Serve with a salad of option.

Notes.

Marinate heart in apple cider vinegar for 24-hour before food preparation, to remove solid blood smell.


Hidden Liver Meatballs.

Components.

•	1 pound ground pork.

•	1 pound US Wellness Meats Liverwurst, cut.

•	Strong fat of choice for frying (pastured lard, bacon fat, duck fat, or tallow).


Directions.

•	In a food processor, incorporate the ground pork and liverwurst until smooth.

- Roll the blend into 1 1/2- inch broad meatballs and also reserved.

- Warmth 1 to 2 tbsps of fat of option in a large stainless steel frying pan over medium warmth. Include meatballs to the frying pan, making sure not to jam-pack (if so, cook in two batches).

- Fry on all sides till browned as well as prepared through, concerning 13 to 15 mins total.

- Get rid of warmth and allow the remainder 5 mins prior to serving with your preferred dipping sauce.

Natural Herb Roasted Bone Marrow.

COMPONENTS.

- Marrow bones from grass-fed/pasture-raised beef, 1-2 each.

- Fresh rosemary.

- Fresh thyme.

- Unrefined salt and black pepper.

DIRECTIONS.

- Marrow is rich, decadent and also elegant. The marrow from one or two bone items suffices for a single person.

- If the bones are frozen, thaw them completely in the refrigerator.

- Preheat the stove to 400 levels. Place the bones in a baking recipe (I baked mine because of mini cast iron pan). Spacing doesn't matter - it can be spaced snugly or freely.

- Carefully cut equivalent parts of fresh rosemary and thyme. I used 1/2 tsp. of sliced herbs for the 4 marrow bones. Sprinkle the natural herbs over the marrow bones.

- Roast for around 15 mins, up until no longer pink inside. You intend to capture them before the marrow starts to "cookout" of the bones.

- Season with salt and pepper and also offer hot. Make use of a spoon to scoop out the marrow.

- Conserve any type of drippings, as well as remaining marrow, in an impermeable container in the fridge for a number of days. I finely chop the remaining marrow as well as throw it with hot, prepared vegetables for a taste and also nutrient boost.

NUTRITION INFO.

Offering dimension: 1-2 marrow bones.

BARBEQUE Chicken Livers and Hearts.

Active ingredients.

•	1 lb chicken hearts - ideal bought from your neighborhood farmer, organic, and also totally free range!

•	1 lb chicken livers, same as above.

•	sea salt.

•	black pepper.

•	bamboo skewers, pre-soaked in water for 1 hr from both sides.

Guidelines.

•	The liver and also hearts could come icy in little packets. Thaw and offer room temperature levels.

•	Now clean both the hearts and also livers from capillaries and also excess fat.

•	The heart's difficult top components can be eliminated with a sharp knife.

- In the meantime, prepare the BBQ - we use just charcoals, yet you can use gas and also bring to med/high warmth.

- Currently thread the hearts on the skewers, 5 to 7 each, relying on their dimension.

- After cleaning the livers, focusing not to damage or smush them, lay flat on a flexible grilling basket.

- Season both liver and hearts with sea salt as well as freshly ground black pepper.

- The livers will stick on the grill otherwise and also easily break apart.

- Now set on the grill and cook till the desired doneness is reached.

- We like our hearts well done, and also the livers still tender.

- Fresh tahini sauce is a fantastic covering for both portions of meat!

## SUMMARY.

Pick Your Favorite Meat For Supper (Or Attempt
Something New).

If you enjoy poultry, you may wish to start with the
bacon-wrapped chicken bites, crispy Indian hen
drumsticks or the slow stove jerk poultry.

Body organ meats are a fantastic option when you 'd
like a budget-friendly supper! Try the rosemary liver
hamburgers or baked bone marrow-- they make certain
to be a hit.

,

# CONCLUSION

While the all meat pattern is still very new, our ancestors from hundreds of years back have actually been following a comparable consuming method, several of which have actually measured up to 100 years old.

With the unbelievable quantity of carnivores revitalizing their health - and also research study to back it up - the carnivore diet will certainly continue to climb in appeal.

Adhering To the Carnivore Diet plan entails consuming just meat, fish, as well as animal products, getting rid of all various other foods. It's claimed to assist weight-loss and a number of health and wellness problems. What's even more, it's high in fat and sodium, has no fiber or helpful plant substances, and is tough to keep long-term.

Many people that have taken on the carnivore diet plan report much faster weight management improved psychological quality, much healthier food digestion, and also even boosted sports performance. I absolutely don't question the unscientific records of individuals that have found a remarkable remedy for debilitating chronic health problems with this diet plan. For a lot of these individuals, absolutely nothing else they had actually attempted worked.

Generally, the Carnivore Diet is needlessly limiting. Consuming a well-balanced diet plan with a selection of healthy and balanced foods is more lasting and also will likely manage you more wellness advantages.

# DISCLAIMER

This book is not intended as a substitute for the medical advice of physicians. The reader should regularly consult a physician in matters relating to his/her health and particularly with respect to any symptoms that may require diagnosis or medical attention.

(diet, health)

# ABOUT THE AUTHOR


**MY NAME IS  ALAN J MORRIS** i am

I really love educating people on how to stay healthy and live the life of their dreams.

**Do Not Go Yet; One Last Thing To Do**

If you enjoyed this book or found it useful, I'd be very grateful if you'd post a short review on Amazon. Your support does make a difference, and I read all the reviews personally so I can get your feedback and make this book even better.

***Thanks again for your support!***